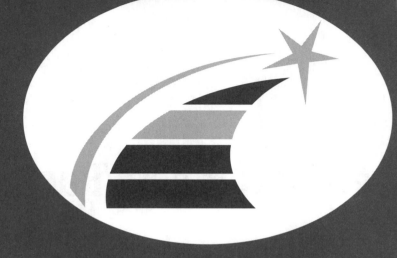

Step 3: Certify

Congratulations on reaching the certification step in your career! As you know, certified coders are in top demand in today's marketplace. That's why, as a lifelong coder and educator, I have dedicated myself to providing the most up-to-date, comprehensive, and user-friendly certification review books on the market. I update this book every year so you will have the best tool possible when studying for your certification exam. It's time to hit the books. *You can do it! I know you can!*

— Carol J. Buck, MS, CPC, CPC-H, CCS-P

Track your progress!

See the checklist in the back of this book to learn more about your next step toward coding success!

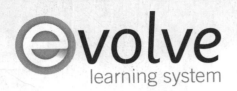
evolve
learning system

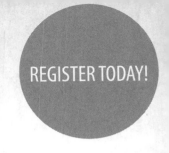

To access your Student Resources, visit:

http://evolve.elsevier.com/Buck/facility

Evolve® Student Resources for *Buck: The Extra Step: Facility-Based Coding Practice* offer the following features:

- ## Study Tips
  Thoughts and advice from the author to help medical coding students.

- ## Content Updates
  The latest content updates from the author to keep you current with recent developments in this area.

- ## WebLinks
  Links to places of interest on the Web, specific to your classroom needs.

- ## HCPCS and ICD-9-CM Updates
  The latest developments and rules for these coding sets.

- ## Rationales for Patient Cases
  In-depth explanations for the correct answers to patient cases.

ELSEVIER

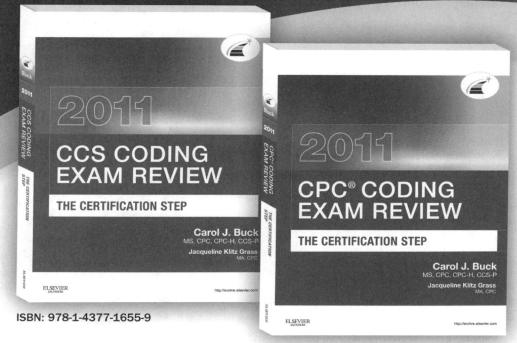

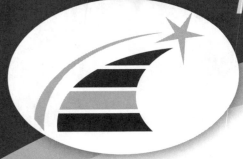
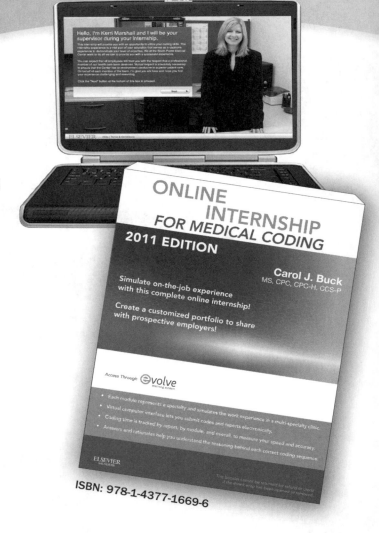

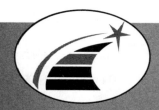

2011

THE EXTRA STEP

FACILITY-BASED CODING PRACTICE

Carol J. Buck
MS, CPC, CPC-H, CCS-P
Program Director, Retired
Medical Secretary Programs
Northwest Technical College
East Grand Forks, Minnesota

Jacqueline Klitz Grass
MA, CPC
Coding Specialist
Grand Forks, North Dakota

ELSEVIER
SAUNDERS

http://evolve.elsevier.com

ELSEVIER
SAUNDERS

3251 Riverport Lane
St. Louis, Missouri 63043

THE EXTRA STEP: FACILITY-BASED CODING PRACTICE

ISBN: 978-1-4377-1659-7

Notices

Knowledge and best practice in this field are constantly changing. As new research and experience broaden our understanding, changes in research methods, professional practices, or medical treatment may become necessary.

Practitioners and researchers must always rely on their own experience and knowledge in evaluating and using any information, methods, compounds, or experiments described herein. In using such information or methods they should be mindful of their own safety and the safety of others, including parties for whom they have a professional responsibility.

With respect to any drug or pharmaceutical products identified, readers are advised to check the most current information provided (i) on procedures featured or (ii) by the manufacturer of each product to be administered, to verify the recommended dose or formula, the method and duration of administration, and contraindications. It is the responsibility of practitioners, relying on their own experience and knowledge of their patients, to make diagnoses, to determine dosages and the best treatment for each individual patient, and to take all appropriate safety precautions.

To the fullest extent of the law, neither the Publisher nor the authors, contributors, or editors, assume any liability for any injury and/or damage to persons or property as a matter of products liability, negligence or otherwise, or from any use or operation of any methods, products, instructions, or ideas contained in the material herein.

NOTE: *Current Procedural Terminology, 2011,* was used in updating this text.

Current Procedural Terminology (CPT) is copyright 2010 American Medical Association. All Rights Reserved. No fee schedules, basic units, relative values, or related listings are included in CPT. The AMA assumes no liability for the data contained herein. Applicable FARS/DFARS restrictions apply to government use.

Library of Congress Cataloging-in-Publication Data

Buck, Carol J.
  The extra step : facility-based coding practice / Carol J. Buck, Jacqueline Klitz Grass.
    p. ; cm.
  ISBN 978-1-4377-1659-7 (pbk. : alk. paper)   1. Nosology—Code numbers—Problems, exercices, etc.   I. Grass, Jacqueline Klitz.   II. Title.
  [DNLM: 1. Forms and Records Control—Problems and Exercises.   2. Medical Records—Problems and Exercises.   3. Terminology as Topic—Problems and Exercises.   W 18.2 B922e 2011]
  RB115.B8247 2011
  616.001′2—dc22   2010024477

Publisher: Michael S. Ledbetter
Associate Developmental Editor: Jennifer Boudreau
Publishing Services Manager: Pat Joiner-Myers
Project Manager: Marlene Weeks
Senior Designer: Amy Buxton

Working together to grow
libraries in developing countries

www.elsevier.com | www.bookaid.org | www.sabre.org

ELSEVIER   BOOK AID International   Sabre Foundation

Printed in the United States of America

Last digit is the print number: 9   8   7   6   5   4   3   2   1

Development of This Edition

This book would not have been possible without a team of educators and professionals, including practicing coders and technical consultants. The combined efforts of the team members have made this text an incredible learning tool.

TEAM LEADER

Jacqueline Klitz Grass, MA, CPC
Coding Specialist
Grand Forks, North Dakota

SENIOR CODING SPECIALIST

Lindsay-Anne Jenkins, CRNA, CPC, CPC-H, CPC-I, CIRCC, CANPC
Coding and Auditing Specialist
St. Louis, Missouri

SENIOR ICD-9-CM AND ICD-10-CM CODING SPECIALIST

Karla R. Lovaasen, RHIA, CCS, CCS-P
Coding and Consulting Services
Abingdon, Maryland

—Coauthor of *ICD-9-CM Coding: Theory and Practice, 2011 Edition*, St. Louis, 2011, Saunders.

SENIOR COLLABORATOR AND ICD-10-CM CONSULTANT

Nancy Maguire, ACS, CRT, PCS, FCS, HCS-D, APC, AFC
Physician Consultant for Auditing and Education
Universal City, Texas

QUERY MANAGER

Patricia Cordy Henricksen, MS, CHCA, CPC-I, CPC, CCP-P, PCS
Approved PMCC Instructor
Education Director, Lexington Local Chapter of AAPC
Bluegrass Medical Managers Association
Lexington, Kentucky

QUERY TEAM

Debra Kroll, RHIT
Denial and Billing Compliance Supervisor
Altru Health System
Grand Forks, North Dakota

Introduction

The skill of medical coding is acquired through many long hours of practice. It is not a skill that can be learned simply by reading about code assignment. Only through a detailed analysis of a wide variety of reports can the coder be proficient. Once you have coded a particular service or diagnosis, you have improved your knowledge base and you will find it is easier the next time you code that particular service or diagnosis. The key words to improve your coding ability are patience and practice.

This product can be used to assist you in improving your coding ability in a specific coding area or for experience in a broad array of specialty areas. Users have found these real-life reports are helpful in preparing for facility certification examinations, such as CPC-H and CCS, because they provide experience in coding many facility services.

The text is composed of 13 chapters:

Chapter	1	Integumentary
Chapter	2	Gastrointestinal
Chapter	3	Nephrology
Chapter	4	Neurology/Neurosurgery
Chapter	5	Obstetric and Gynecologic Surgery and Ophthalmology
Chapter	6	Orthopedic
Chapter	7	Otorhinolaryngology
Chapter	8	General Surgery
Chapter	9	Emergency Department
Chapter	10	Diagnostic Radiology
Chapter	11	Interventional Radiology, Radiation Oncology, and Nuclear Medicine
Chapter	12	Cardiology
Chapter	13	Inpatient Cases

There are a variable number of reports within each chapter to give you experience in each of these major coding areas. This edition features abstracting questions presented at the end of each report. These questions will assist you as you improve your critical thinking skills necessary to code medical reports. Your instructor has access to these answers via the Evolve website. Students not enrolled in a course do not have access to these answers.

Contents

List of Physicians

Rush K. Peterson, MD	Allergy & Immunology
Janice E. Larson, MD	Anesthesia
James Noonar, MD	Cardiology
Marvin Elhart, MD	Cardiology
David Barton, MD	Cardiothoracic Surgery
Robert Brown, MD	Critical Care
Elmer Lauer, MD	Dermatology
Noah Lovejoy, MD	Dermatology
Laddie N. Noss, MD	Diabetes & Internal Medicine
Paul Sutton, MD	Emergency Medicine—**Hospital Employee**
Gordon Jayco, MD	Endocrinology
Phil Doron, MD	Endocrinology
Frank Gaul, MD	Family Practice
Daniel G. Olanka, MD	Gastroenterology
Larry P. Friendly, MD	Gastroenterology
Gary I. Sanchez, MD	General Surgery
Loren White, MD	General Surgery
Gerald Lorabi, MD	Hematology
Lou Lin, MD	Infectious Diseases
Alma Naraquist, MD	Internal Medicine
Ronald Green, MD	Internal Medicine and Critical Care
Leslie Alanda, MD	Internal Medicine and Vascular
Edward Riddle, MD	Interventional Radiology
Monica J. Hamilton, MD	Interventional Radiology
George Orbitz, MD	Nephrology
Gordon Jayco, MD	Nephrology
Timothy L. Pleasant, MD	Neurology
Jerome Nelson, MD	Neurophysiology
Phillip Hart, MD	Neuroradiology—**Hospital Employee**
Alfa Aljabar, MD	Nuclear Medicine
Andy Martinez, MD	Obstetrics & Gynecology
Rapheal White, MD	Oncology
Rita Wimer, MD	Ophthalmology
Mohomad Almaz, MD	Orthopedics
Jeff King, MD	Otorhinolaryngology
Grey Lonewolf, MD	Pathology
Rolando Ortez, MD	Pediatrics & Neonatology
Mary Barneswell, MD	Physical Therapy
Mark Erickson, MD	Plastic Surgery
Samuel Warner, MD	Podiatry
James Eagle, MD	Radiation Oncology
Morton Monson, MD	Radiology
Gregory Dawson, MD	Respiratory Care
John Hodgson, MD	Surgical Neurosurgery
Ronald Ripple, MD	Thoracic Surgery
Ira Avila, MD	Urology
Paula Smithson, MD	Urology

Technical and Professional Components

Many codes have a technical and professional component. For example, most radiology codes have a technical component (-TC) and a professional component (-26). The Centers for Medicare and Medicaid Services (CMS) annually develops a list of codes with technical and professional components and each component has a specified reimbursement amount. Hospital facility services are reported on a UB-04 Universal Health Insurance Claim Form. The UB-04 is used to report only the "technical component" of services; therefore, the -TC modifier is not required. If the hospital facility employs a physician, the physician's services would usually be reported on the CMS-1500 Health Insurance Claim Form.

If you were a coder for an outpatient clinic, you would report services on the CMS-1500. If you reported a physician service with a code that had a professional and a technical component, you would report that service with modifier -26 if only the professional portion of the service was provided. For example, if a clinic physician went to the hospital and supervised and then interpreted an x-ray followed by a written report, you would report the physician's component on a CMS-1500 with a modifier -26 and the hospital facility would report the technical component of the x-ray on the UB-04 with no modifier. If you were reporting only the technical component of a service provided at the clinic, you would report the service on a CMS-1500 and would add the -TC modifier to the service code. If the code had a technical and professional component and your facility provided both components, you would submit the code with no modifier, thereby reporting both the technical and professional components.

On the job, you will be provided with a list of the codes that have the technical and professional components and you would refer to the list to determine which codes were to be submitted with the -TC or -26 modifier. Within this text, you are reporting the hospital facility services, which would be reported on the UB-04 and will therefore not require the -TC modifier.

Chapter 1
Integumentary

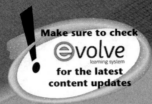

Make sure to check
evolve learning system
for the latest
content updates

Case 1: Excision, Basal Cell Carcinoma

LOCATION: Outpatient, Hospital

PATIENT: Dana Kelley

PREOPERATIVE DIAGNOSIS: Basal cell carcinoma, right side of nose.

POSTOPERATIVE DIAGNOSIS: Same.

SURGICAL FINDINGS: Healing 5-mm ulcer, right side of nose, with surrounding inflammatory response.

SURGICAL PROCEDURE: Excision of basal cell carcinoma, right side of nose, with reconstruction by 3 × 2.5 cm bi-lobed flap.

SURGEON: Gary Sanchez, MD

ANESTHESIA: Standby sedation with 5 cc of 1% Xylocaine with 1:100,000 epinephrine.

DESCRIPTION OF PROCEDURE: The patient's face was prepped with Betadine scrub and solution, and draped in a routine sterile fashion. The lesion and the surrounding tissue for the flap were both anesthetized with a total of 5 cc of 1% Xylocaine with 1:100,000 epinephrine. The lesion was excised circumferentially with a 5-mm margin. It was submitted for frozen section with a tag on the inferior aspect. The lesion was clear on all margins. Bleeding was electrocoagulated. We developed a 3 × 2.5 cm bilobed flap based on the left side, rotating it in place and insetting it with 5–0 Prolene. Antibiotic ointment and Surgicel were applied followed by a 4 × 4. The patient tolerated the procedure well and left the area in good condition.

Pathology Report Later Indicated: Malignant lesion (basal cell carcinoma).

CPT Code(s): 14060 Excision, transfer (by size in the case, under 10mm)

ICD-9-CM Code(s): 173.3 neoplasm, nose, external

ICD-10-CM Code(s): _____

Abstracting Questions

1. Is the lesion intranasal (within the nose) or external nose? _External_

2. Was the repair done with an adjacent tissue transfer or free graft? _Adj. tissue transfer_

3. Are the excision and repair both reported? _No_

(Answers to all Abstracting Questions are located on your Instructor's Evolve site. If you are not currently enrolled in a course, you will not have access to these answers. Record your responses to these questions and ask your instructor for the answers.)

Case 2: Ulcer Repair

OPERATIVE REPORT

LOCATION: Outpatient, Hospital

PATIENT: Andy Green

PREOPERATIVE DIAGNOSES
1. Chronic ulcer of the left ischium.
2. Status post debridement of left ischial ulcer.

POSTOPERATIVE DIAGNOSES: Same.

SURGICAL FINDINGS: Approximately 8-cm diameter open wound, left ischium with large clot.

SURGICAL PROCEDURE: Minimal debridement, left ischial ulcer with complex closure.

SURGEON: Gary Sanchez, MD

ANESTHESIA: General endotracheal.

hip

DESCRIPTION OF PROCEDURE: The patient was intubated and turned in the prone position, the ischial area was prepped with Betadine scrub and solution, and draped in routine sterile fashion. Following preparation of Betadine scrub and solution, the old clot was removed from the wound and more necrotic tissue was removed. The wound was closed in layers with interrupted 2–0 Monocryl and interrupted 0 Prolene for the skin using vertical mattress sutures. A #10 Jackson-Pratt drain was placed at the wound and brought out through a separate stab wound incision. It was sutured to the wound with 0 Prolene. Tegaderm was applied to the actual wound itself to prevent fecal contamination; Kerlix fluffs were placed on top of this with an Elastoplast dressing. Estimated blood loss was negligible. The patient tolerated the procedure well and left the area in good condition.

Pathology Report Later Indicated: Benign tissue.

CPT Code(s): _13101 repair add 5cm   13102 repair, ulcer, complex_

ICD-9-CM Code(s): _707.8 Ulcer, hip_

ICD-10-CM Code(s): _____

Abstracting Questions

1. Are the excision and repair both reported? __no__
2. Was the repair simple, intermediate, or complex? __Complex__
3. Does the size of the wound affect the coding? __yes__
4. How many codes are required to report the total size? __2__
5. How does the location of the wound repair affect coding? __coded on "trunk" by location or hip__

Case 3: Ulcer Debridement

OPERATIVE REPORT

LOCATION: Outpatient, Hospital

PATIENT: Eric Crest

PREOPERATIVE DIAGNOSIS: Large necrotic pressure ulcer of the right lateral leg.

POSTOPERATIVE DIAGNOSIS: Large necrotic pressure ulcer of the right lateral leg.

SURGEON: Gary Sanchez, MD

PROCEDURE: Sharp debridement of soft tissues, tendon, and fascia down to muscle of the right lateral leg. Measures approximately 4–5 cm in length × 3 cm in width × 1 cm in depth.

DESCRIPTION OF PROCEDURE: He basically has no sensation in his lower extremities. Then using sharp dissection, we sharply debrided all the necrotic tissue. This included some tendinous tissues. This was down into some muscle in a couple of spots. This was getting down to fairly close to the fibular head. There was not a lot of tissue between here and the fibular head. We debrided all the necrotic tissue. There were a few areas along the periphery that actually had hypergranulation tissue. These were treated with silver nitrate. Hemostasis was achieved. We ended up with a fair amount of necrotic debris and things cleaned up pretty well here. Could be looking at placing a TransiGel dressing at this time. The patient tolerated the procedure well.

Pathology Report Later Indicated: Benign ulcerative tissue.

CPT Code(s): 11043 debridement, muscle.

ICD-9-CM Code(s): 707.24 707.09 Ulcer, decubitus

ICD-10-CM Code(s): _____

Abstracting Questions

1. Was a repair documented for this procedure? _no_

2. How deep of level was documented for the debridement—skin, subcutaneous tissue, muscle fascia, muscle, or bone? _Muscle_

3. When referencing the Index of the ICD-9-CM for pressure ulcer as the diagnosis, you are directed to:
   Ulcer decubitus, other

Case 4: Dressing Change

OPERATIVE REPORT

LOCATION: Outpatient, Hospital

PATIENT: Larry Knight

PREOPERATIVE DIAGNOSIS: Sartorius flap with wound vac to the right groin.

POSTOPERATIVE DIAGNOSIS: Same.

SURGEON: Gary Sanchez, MD

PROCEDURE PERFORMED: Wound vac dressing change.

INDICATIONS: The patient has a wound vac that has been placed for management of his wound in his right groin. This is status post sartorius flap.

DESCRIPTION OF PROCEDURE: The patient was premedicated with 5 mg of morphine IV. The wound vac was discontinued. The dressing was removed. The wound was nice and clean. This was extracting in and filling in nicely. A new small sponge was cut to the size and shape of the groin wound. The surrounding areas were cleaned. This had been draped off sterilely prior to this. Sponges were applied to the wound, and saline retaining dressing was applied over this. A small hole was made on top of the sponge. Vacuum tubing was inserted in this. This was attached to the saline retaining dressing. This was then connected to wound vac. This was placed at 125 mm Mercury of pressure. This sealed down nice. This contracted in well. The patient tolerated the procedure well. Dressing changes were also obtained off his right foot and left heel. The left heel looked fine. The dressing will remain off and we will place a Duoderm on this. The wound has an eschar that is developing over this. We will use Duoderm on this for now. His right heel and the small one on the medial side of the top foot looks good, these are nice and clean. The large one over the lateral top part of the right foot shows granulation around the periphery; however, the central aspect shows fibrinous exudate and questionable viability of tissue. This again goes rather deep.

The dressing will remain off. We will start having him go to whirlpool twice a day and collagenase this twice a day. *Therapy attention*

CPT Code(s): *97605 wound, neg pressure therapy*

ICD-9-CM Code(s): *attention, surgical dressing V58.31*

ICD-10-CM Code(s): _____

Abstracting Questions

1. Was there anything more than dressing change on the groin wound? *Yes*

2. How is the management of the right and left foot wounds reported? _____

3. How would the code be located in the CPT index for this dressing change? *Wound negative pressure therapy*

4. The size of the wound is not documented. How does this affect coding? *code smallest wound repair*

5. How is the diagnosis code located in the Index of the ICD-9-CM? *attention to, surg. dressing*
not reported seperately b/c dressings removed at same time?

Case 5: Split Thickness Skin Graft

OPERATIVE REPORT

LOCATION: Outpatient, Hospital

PATIENT: Manny Hartwell

PREOPERATIVE DIAGNOSES
1. Ulcer of the right lateral foot.
2. Superficial ulcer of the right anterior ankle.

POSTOPERATIVE DIAGNOSES: Same.

SURGEON: Gary Sanchez, MD

PROCEDURES PERFORMED
1. Split thickness skin graft to right lateral foot, 7 cm × 5 cm.
2. Split thickness skin graft to right anterior ankle ulcer, 2 cm × 3 cm.

INDICATIONS: The patient is a 75-year-old male who has developed wounds to his feet. He has been revascularized. These wounds have started to show signs of healing. The main concern was on the right lateral foot. He also developed an ulcer to the anterior ankle. We examined this today in the holding room before surgery and this wound was also clean, but it sloughed off the epithelialization of the skin/blister over this. I recommended to him that we also skin graft this at the same time. We discussed the procedure again. We reviewed the risks again. He understands and wishes to proceed with this.

ANESTHESIA: General.

PROCEDURE: This was done under a general anesthetic. The right lateral foot and right anterior ankle wound sites were prepped and debrided of the granulation. There was fair bleeding but neurovascularization of bleeding underneath this. The beds were cleaned. The skin graft was then taken from his right anterior thigh using a dermatome set at 0.012 inch. This was meshed at a ratio of 1:1.5. The one segment that was raised was used to cover both of the wound sites. These were stapled in place and Adaptic, gauze, mineral oil, wet cotton batting, and Fluffs were applied over this and secured in place with an Ace wrap in a snug but not tight manner. He has a small superficial heel ulcer, which was covered with a wet-to-dry dressing, and this was also covered with the above dressing. The patient tolerated the procedure well and went to the recovery room in stable condition.

CPT Code(s): _15120 Split-thickness graft_

ICD-9-CM Code(s): _707.13 foot_　　　　　　　　_707.17 ankle_

ICD-10-CM Code(s): _____

Abstracting Questions

1. How are the two separate areas on the right foot and ankle reported? _seperate_
2. How do the measurements of each wound affect code selection? _added together_
3. Is the wet-to-dry dressing applied to the small, superficial heel ulcer reported separately? _no_
4. Are diagnosis codes required for both areas? _yes_

Case 6: Flap with Debridement

OPERATIVE REPORT

LOCATION: Outpatient, Hospital

PATIENT: Kenneth Osborne

PREOPERATIVE DIAGNOSES
1. Sartorius flap to the right groin with wound vac management of the wound.
2. Large, nonhealing wounds of the right foot with an area of eschar.
3. Heel ulcer of left foot.

POSTOPERATIVE DIAGNOSES
1. Sartorius flap to the right groin with wound vac management of the wound.
2. Large, nonhealing wounds of the right foot with an area of eschar.
3. Heel ulcer of left foot.

SURGEON: Gary Sanchez, MD

PROCEDURES PERFORMED
1. Wound vac dressing change. 97605
2. Debridement of right foot.
3. Debridement of left heel ulcer.

INDICATION: The patient is a 54-year-old male whom we have done a sartorius flap on. He has been using wound vac for management of this wound. This has been going well. We have been using Tender wet dressing change on his right foot. He has also developed a heel ulcer somehow, even though he is on a Clinitron bed, of his left heel. We will debride this area, as well as the eschar on his right foot.

DESCRIPTION OF PROCEDURE: The patient was given 5 mg of morphine IV prior to the start of the procedure. We took down the old sponge dressing in the right groin. We disconnected the wound tubing and the machine had been placed on standby. The wound was inspected and was nice and clean, and it continues to contract in. We sterilely draped off the area and cut a new small sponge to the right size. We placed this and secured in place with a retaining drape. A small hole was cut on the top of the sponge and a suction tube was inserted through this. This was secured in place with another retaining dressing. We connected it to the wound vac and placed it at 125 mm of continuous suction; this had a good seal. The sponge contracted out nicely. We then removed the dressing from his right foot. He had eschar over the top portion of the foot. This was thin in the periphery but was rather thick and deep in the more central aspect. We sharply debrided this back with 19 sq cm debrided. We still were not down to bone after debriding this, but we did debride muscle. Some of this area looks viable underneath, but some of this is questionable at best. At this time, though, we will continue with the dressing changes and see what comes of this yet. New Tender wet dressings were applied.

On the left heel he had developed a 10 sq cm superficial ulcer. It had started draining as he had a hole in the "blister." We debrided this blister open. He has one area that does appear to be maybe a little bit deeper, but we will just put Tender wet dressings on this also for now.

We will then probably look at Duoderm down the road. I think this part should do fine with some good local match. We will just have to continue to watch this for now.

Pathology Report Later Indicated: Benign ulcerative tissue.

CPT Code(s): _11043, 11042_   97605 wound therapy

ICD-9-CM Code(s): _ulcer 707.15 707.14_

ICD-10-CM Code(s): _____

Abstracting Questions

1. Are the debridements for the foot and heel reported separately? _yes_

Case 7: Lesion Excision

OPERATIVE REPORT

LOCATION: Outpatient, Hospital

PATIENT: Dave Schroeder

INDICATIONS: This patient has a mole of the left chest wall that has been changing in character for the past two months. When we saw this in the office, it was originally dark with surrounding erythema, but now it has lost some of its pigmentation. Nevertheless, there is still a definite lesion present.

PREOPERATIVE DIAGNOSIS: Changing compound nevus of the left chest wall.

POSTOPERATIVE DIAGNOSIS: Pending.

SURGEON: Gary Sanchez, MD

SURGICAL FINDINGS: A 5-mm diameter, lightly pigmented lesion on the left lateral chest wall, benign.

SURGICAL PROCEDURE: Excision of lesion of left chest wall with 5-mm proximal and distal margins and 2-mm lateral margins.

ANESTHESIA: 1% Xylocaine and 1:100,000 Epinephrine, 3 cc.

DESCRIPTION OF PROCEDURE: Chest wall was prepped in Betadine solution and draped in sterile fashion. The lesion was anesthetized with a total of 3 cc of 1% Xylocaine and 1:100,000 epinephrine. The lesion was excised elliptically with 5-mm proximal and distal margins and 2-mm lateral margins. Bleeding was electrocoagulated. The wound was closed with subcuticular 4–0 Monocryl in interrupted twists of 4–0 Monocryl. Steri-Strips were applied. The patient tolerated the procedure well and left the area in good condition.

Pathology Report Later Indicated: Benign tissue.

CPT Code(s): _11402 Excision, benign lesion_

ICD-9-GM Code(s): _216.5 neoplasm, skin, chest (wall), benign_

ICD-10-CM Code(s): _____

Abstracting Questions

1. Does the benign/malignant status of excised lesion affect code selection? _benign "yes"_

2. Does the size of the lesion affect code selection? _yes_

3. Does the location on the body affect code selection? _yes_

4. Does the number of lesions affect code selection? _no_

5. Preoperative diagnosis is listed as nevus of chest wall. How is this diagnosis affected by the final pathological outcome? _it supports the pre-op diagnosis_

Case 8: Incision and Drainage

OPERATIVE REPORT

LOCATION: Outpatient, Hospital

PATIENT: John Wellington

PROCEDURE: Incision and drainage

SURGEON: Loren White, MD

INDICATION: This is a 23-year-old male being admitted for abscesses and lymphangitis of the left arm. He has two small pustules on the left hand, one on the radial side of the proximal phalanx of the fourth finger and the other in the web space between the fourth and fifth fingers.

PROCEDURE NOTE: The areas were cleansed with alcohol, 1% lidocaine with bicarb, infiltrated locally, and the wounds cleaned with Betadine prep. A #11 blade was used to make a cross incision. Not much pus was found. The wounds were quite superficial. The wound was expanded by cutting out small corners of the incision to allow for further drainage. Antibiotic ointment and a gauze and Kling dressing were applied.

ASSESSMENT: 1. Pustule. 2. Abscess. 3. Lymphangitis, left arm.

PLAN: The patient will be admitted to the hospital for IV antibiotic therapy. Wound cultures are pending.

_25025_ ?

Pathology Report Later Indicated: Benign tissue and culture.

CPT Code(s): _10061_ _Drainage, skin, incision/drainage of abcess, mult._
ICD-9-CM Code(s): _686.9_ _682.3 Abcess, arm_
ICD-10-CM Code(s): _Pustule_

Abstracting Questions

1. Does the type of lesion affect the code selection? _yes_
2. What other criteria affect code selection? _body part, size, location, how many_

Chapter 2
Gastrointestinal

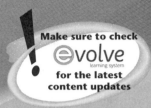

Make sure to check **evolve** learning system for the latest content updates

Case 9: Sigmoidoscopy

OPERATIVE REPORT

LOCATION: Outpatient, Hospital

PATIENT: Lorretta Hatfield

PREOPERATIVE DIAGNOSIS: Diarrhea.

POSTOPERATIVE DIAGNOSIS: Mild resolving patchy colitis, nonspecific, probably infectious. The patient should still be worked up for fever as the colitis may not be the cause of the fever.

SURGEON: Larry Friendly, MD

PROCEDURE PERFORMED: Flexible sigmoidoscopy.

INDICATIONS: 42-year-old white female with SLE and chronic renal failure on hemodialysis who has had diarrhea since returning from her vacation where she was hospitalized. Her stools were negative. She did well, but on the day of discharge she began having diarrhea again and was readmitted today. She has had only one stool within the last four hours. The stools mostly seem to be nocturnal. She has had no antibiotics recently, no one else is ill.

FINDINGS: The Pentax videosigmoidoscope was inserted without difficulty to 50 cm. Careful inspection of the mid and distal descending, sigmoid, and rectum revealed patchy erythema, minimal friability, and some mild edema. There was no discrete ulceration, no exudate. No biopsies were obtained. The patient tolerated the procedure well.

IMPRESSION: Mild patchy colitis that appears to be resolving, consistent with infectious colitis.

PLAN: The diarrhea is slowly resolving and probably will resolve spontaneously. We will check the stools but no treatment for now unless she continues to be symptomatic; if so, I would give her ciprofloxacin.

CPT Code(s): _45330 Sig. exploration_

ICD-9-CM Code(s): _009.0 Col. 780.60 Fev._

ICD-10-CM Code(s): _____

Abstracting Questions

1. Does the documentation support the extent of exam for a sigmoidoscopy, according to CPT definition?

    yes

2. Does the designation of flexible affect code selection? _yes_

3. Does the fact that "no biopsies" were taken affect code selection? _yes_

4. What does SLE stand for? _Systemic Lupus Erythmatosus_

5. Can you define the following terms from this case? _____

    a. Erythema _Redness of the skin_

    b. Friability _brittle_

    c. Edema _Swelling due to excess fluids_

    d. Exudate _Discharge_

Case 10: Colonoscopy

OPERATIVE REPORT

LOCATION: Outpatient, Hospital

PATIENT: Greg Davis

PROCEDURE: Colonoscopy with multiple biopsies.

PREOPERATIVE DIAGNOSIS: Rule out cytomegalovirus colitis.

POSTOPERATIVE DIAGNOSIS: Mild patchy erythema in the descending, sigmoid, and rectum, nonspecific, not characteristic of colitis.

SURGEON: Daniel Olanka, MD

INDICATION: This is a 28-year-old white male with pancreatic and kidney transplant secondary to diabetes that presents with one week of diarrhea, abdominal cramping, and nausea and vomiting. He was treated with ganciclovir, for presumed CMV enteritis based on rising CMV serology. He was not seen, however, by anyone. He presents now dehydrated and with creatinine of 3.1. The procedure is indicated to rule out CMV colitis.

PREOPERATIVE MEDICATION: Demerol 50 mg IV, Versed 4 mg IV.

FINDINGS: The Pentax video colonoscope was inserted easily into the cecum. Ileocecal valve was identified, and the appendiceal orifice was seen. The terminal ileum was entered a distance of 5 cm. No lesions were seen. Inspection of the cecum, ascending colon, hepatic flexure, transverse colon, and splenic flexure revealed no erythema, ulceration, exudate, and friability in the mucosa. Biopsies were obtained in the right colon of normal mucosa. The distal descending, sigmoid, and rectum revealed patchy erythema without ulceration, no friability, and really no loss of vascular pattern. There were just erythematous areas, nonspecific. Biopsies were obtained of these areas also. The patient tolerated the procedure well.

IMPRESSION: Nonspecific mild erythema in the distal descending, sigmoid, and rectum, not characteristic of CMV colitis, biopsied normal terminal ileum, normal colon otherwise.

PLAN: Esophagogastroduodenoscopy.

Pathology Report Later Indicated: Benign tissue.

CPT Code(s): _45380_

ICD-9-CM Code(s): _787.91   784.00   787.01_

ICD-10-CM Code(s): _Diarrhea   Cramps   Nausea w/ vom_

Abstracting Questions

1. Does the extent of the exam support the reporting of a colonoscopy? _yes_
2. What was done to indicate if this was diagnostic or more extensive? _biopsies_
3. Since the colonoscopy was "normal," what diagnosis code(s) is/are reported? _symptoms_
4. What does CMV stand for? _Cytomegalovirus_
5. Is the status post kidney and pancreas transplant reported? _no_

Case 11: Esophagogastroduodenoscopy

OPERATIVE REPORT

LOCATION: Outpatient, Hospital

PATIENT: George Hall

PREOPERATIVE DIAGNOSIS: Upper gastrointestinal bleed.   *Endo*

POSTOPERATIVE DIAGNOSIS: Diffuse gastric mucosal lesions.

SURGEON: Larry Friendly, MD

PROCEDURE PERFORMED: Esophagogastroduodenoscopy.

HISTORY: The patient presented with a four-day history of black tarry stools. He has a previous history of cirrhosis secondary to drinking. He has also had a stroke. The risks of the procedure were explained in detail to him. The patient said he is aware of this. He had an endoscopy similar to this a number of years ago, but he does not remember the results.

PROCEDURE: After obtaining consent, his throat was sprayed with Xylocaine spray. He was given 2 mg of Versed and 50 of fentanyl and was monitored during the procedure. An IV of Ringer's lactate was started on this gentleman because of his history.

After adequate sedation and placement of a bite block, the therapeutic endoscope was placed into the esophagus easily under direct vision. The gentleman has a small hiatus hernia, but no varices. On entering the stomach, in the proximal stomach there are some gastric mucosal changes, but in the main body and particularly the antrum of the stomach, there is extensive erythematous change consistent with severe gastritis. The duodenum was entered and the bulb has a few areas of duodenitis, but there is no ulceration in the area and there is no problem distal to this area. Bile is seen coming from the papilla. The scope was withdrawn, and the main fundus was evaluated with retroflexed technique. This also has a few punctate changes of gastritis. Biopsies were taken from the antral area in several locations and sent for *H. pylori*. Scope was then withdrawn with the air used to insufflate the stomach and aspirated as we approached the GE-junction. The patient tolerated the procedure without any problems. Patient and daughter were informed of the findings.

Pathology Report Later Indicated: Benign tissue.

CPT Code(s): _____43239_____

ICD-9-CM Code(s): __535.51_____432.39____

ICD-10-CM Code(s): _____

Abstracting Questions

1. Where does the CPT index direct you when you reference in the index for esophagogastroduodenoscopy?
   Endoscopy, GI, Upper

2. Was there a definitive finding upon examination of the stomach? _yes_

Case 12: Flexible Sigmoidoscopy

OPERATIVE REPORT

LOCATION: Outpatient, Hospital

PATIENT: Brian Wright

PREOPERATIVE DIAGNOSIS: Hemoccult-positive stool. Mild anemia.

POSTOPERATIVE DIAGNOSIS: Normal flexible sigmoidoscopy with a moderate number of diverticula in the descending and sigmoid colon.

SURGEON: Daniel Olanka, MD

INDICATION: This is a 46-year-old white male who has Hemoccult-positive stool and hemoglobin of 12.3 with a normal MCV. There is a history of cirrhosis due to alcoholism. He has thrombocytopenia of 49,000. He also has end-stage renal disease on hemodialysis. Given his multiple medical problems, we believed that he would be better served by having a flexible sigmoidoscopy and barium enema.

PREOPERATIVE MEDICATION: None.

FINDINGS: The Pentax video sigmoidoscope was inserted without difficulty to 55 cm. Careful inspection in the mid descending, distal descending, sigmoid, and rectum revealed no erythema, ulceration, exudate, friability, or other mucosal abnormalities. There was a moderate number of diverticula in the descending and sigmoid colon. The patient tolerated the procedure well.

IMPRESSION: Diverticulosis.

PLAN: Patient will receive barium enema. Full report will follow afterward. Patient may need to be endoscoped from above to rule out varices, if this has not been done, if we wish to be aggressive about this.

CPT Code(s): _____ 45330 _____

ICD-9-CM Code(s): ___ 562.10 _____ 792.1 ____ 258.9 _____

ICD-10-CM Code(s): ___ 1 _____ ↓ _____ ↓ _____
                        Div.   Stool   polyglandular dis

Abstracting Questions

1. Is it appropriate to continue to report the presenting symptoms as diagnoses? __ yes _____

Case 13: Colonoscopy through Colostomy

OPERATIVE REPORT

LOCATION: Outpatient, Hospital

PATIENT: Curtis Greenwall

PREOPERATIVE DIAGNOSIS: Gastrointestinal bleeding.

POSTOPERATIVE DIAGNOSIS: Normal colonoscopy.

SURGEON: Daniel Olanka, MD

PROCEDURE PERFORMED: Colonoscopy through colostomy.

INDICATION: This is a 59-year-old white male who was admitted with gastrointestinal bleeding with melenic stool for two days. Hemoglobin was 6, INR 4. He has been given fresh frozen plasma and vitamin K. He was on aspirin, Plavix, and Coumadin. The patient was endoscoped, and there was some superficial gastric ulceration, not bleeding. We were not confident that this was the cause for the patient's blood loss. Therefore, yesterday, he underwent a barium enema; however, the barium enema showed just above the cecum in the ascending colon a spastic area that did not open. I reviewed the films; this looked like spasm and not stricture, but the radiology department was concerned about the potential of this being a malignant stricture.

PREOPERATIVE MEDICATION: Gentamicin 1.5 mg/kg IV and ampicillin 2 grams IV.

PROCEDURE: The Pentax video colonoscope was inserted through the colostomy with no difficulty. The endoscope was rapidly advanced to the cecum. The ileocecal valve was identified and the appendiceal orifice was seen. There was barium coating the mucosa and small lesions could be missed, but certainly any lesion larger than 1 cm or lesions such as strictures would be visualized. Inspection of the cecum, ascending colon, hepatic flexure, transverse colon, splenic flexure, descending colon, and sigmoid colon revealed no erythema, ulceration, exudate, friability, or other mucosal abnormalities. The patient tolerated the procedure well.

IMPRESSION: Normal colonoscopy.

PLAN: The patient will be observed and probably can be discharged any time as long as his hemoglobin remains stable.

CPT Code(s): ___44388 Col. Exp___

ICD-9-CM Code(s): ___578.9___

ICD-10-CM Code(s): _____

Bleed, Gastr

Abstracting Questions

1. Does the access route through the colostomy affect code assignment? ___yes___

2. Because the result of the colonoscopy is documented as normal, what is reported as the diagnosis?

   ___Gastrointestinal bleeding___

Case 14: Colonoscopy with Polypectomy

OPERATIVE REPORT

LOCATION: Outpatient, Hospital

PATIENT: Jackson White

PREOPERATIVE DIAGNOSIS: History of polyp.

POSTOPERATIVE DIAGNOSES
1. Sigmoid carcinoma, approximately 4 cm, at about 18 cm.
2. A small, 2- to 3-mm polyp of the ascending colon, and a 3- to 4-mm sessile polyp in the mid-transverse colon, hot biopsied.

SURGEON: Daniel Olanka, MD

INDICATION: This is a 61-year-old white male who was referred for colonoscopy. The patient had a large pedunculated polyp in the mid-descending colon removed; he continues to have some hematochezia.

PREOPERATIVE MEDICATIONS: Fentanyl 100 mcg IV; Versed 3 mg IV.

FINDINGS: The Pentax video colonoscope was inserted without difficulty to the cecum. The ileocecal valve was identified. The appendiceal orifice was seen. Careful inspection in the cecum revealed no lesions. Inspection of the ascending colon revealed a small 2- to 3-mm polyp. This was hot biopsied. The hepatic flexure was normal. The mid-transverse colon revealed a 3- to 4-mm sessile polyp. This was hot biopsied. The splenic flexure and descending colon revealed no lesions. There were moderate numbers of diverticula in the descending sigmoid colon. In the sigmoid colon, at about 18 cm, was a large 4-cm sessile mass, with friability and some ulceration. Multiple biopsies were obtained. The patient tolerated the procedure well.

IMPRESSION
1. A large 4-cm sessile mass in the sigmoid colon, at 18 cm, consistent with adenocarcinoma.
2. Two small polyps in the proximal colon, removed.
3. Moderate diverticula.

PLAN: The patient will be referred to surgery.

Pathology Report Later Indicated: Malignant neoplasm, sigmoid colon; benign polyps, ascending colon.

CPT Code(s): _45384   removal polyps_

ICD-9-CM Code(s): _153.1   211.3_

ICD-10-CM Code(s): _mal. 19. col   lg int ben_

Abstracting Questions

1. Does the method of polyp removal affect code selection? _yes_
2. Was a single biopsy or multiple biopsies performed? _Mult_
3. Are the malignancy and polyps both reported as diagnoses? _yes_

Case 15: Colonoscopy with Polypectomy

OPERATIVE REPORT

LOCATION: Outpatient, Hospital

PATIENT: Mark Hall

INDICATION: Colon polyps noted on screening flexible sigmoidoscopy.

POSTOPERATIVE DIAGNOSES
1. Colon polyps.
2. Diverticular disease.

SCOPE USED: Pentax video colonoscope.

SURGEON: Daniel Olanka, MD

PREOPERATIVE MEDICATIONS: Demerol 50 mg IV; Versed 3 mg IV.

Informed consent was obtained after the patient was explained the risks, benefits, and alternatives to the procedure.

PHYSICAL EXAMINATION: Blood pressure is 163/82. Pulse is 58. Abdomen is nondistended and nontender. Neurologic: The patient is alert and oriented. No focal signs. Lungs are clear to auscultation. Respirations are unlabored. Coronary: Regular rate and rhythm.

FINDINGS: The scope was passed under direct vision and advanced through the colon to the cecum. The ileocecal valve and appendiceal orifice were well visualized. The cecum, ascending colon, and transverse colon were all found to be normal. There was moderately severe diverticular disease in the descending and sigmoid colon. There was a very large, 3-cm pedunculated mass in the mid-descending colon. Most of this was removed by snare electrocautery. The rest of the rather broad base of the polyp was then injected with saline and again removed by snare technique. The rest of the descending colon was normal. In the sigmoid colon, there was a 5-mm sessile polyp removed by hot biopsy. Sigmoid colon is otherwise unremarkable. Rectum was normal.

IMPRESSION
1. Mid-descending colon polyp measuring approximately 3 cm in diameter. This was removed by piecemeal by snare electrocautery after the base of the polyp was injected with saline.
2. Five-millimeter sessile polyp of the sigmoid colon removed by hot biopsy.
3. Moderately severe diverticular disease.

RECOMMENDATIONS
1. Follow up the results of the biopsy to ensure that there is no invasion of the stock of the polyp. Repeat the biopsies. There was no stock invasion. Next colonoscopy in three years' time.
2. Metamucil or Citrucel one tablespoon daily for diverticular disease.
3. The patient education and handout on diverticular disease.

Pathology Report Later Indicated: Benign tissue.

CPT Code(s): 45385, 45384-59

ICD-9-CM Code(s): 562.10   211.3

ICD-10-CM Code(s):

Abstracting Questions

1. What techniques were used in this case for polyp removal? _Snave & hot biopsy_

Case 16: Esophagogastroduodenoscopy (EGD)

OPERATIVE REPORT

LOCATION: Outpatient, Hospital

PATIENT: Byron Phillips

PREOPERATIVE DIAGNOSIS: Abnormal upper GI (gastrointestinal).

POSTOPERATIVE DIAGNOSIS: Normal endoscopy; 2-cm hiatal hernia.

SURGEON: Daniel Olanka, MD

PROCEDURE PERFORMED: Esophagogastroduodenoscopy.

INDICATION: This is a 59-year-old white male who has had 12 weeks of sore throat. When obtaining an upper GI, he had significant reflux but also aspirated in the left bronchus. He subsequently had undergone video pharyngography, showing significant transfer-type dysphagia. During that study they also apparently saw some increased gastric folds and some abnormality in the distal esophagus. The patient has had a CT of the brainstem, unremarkable. He does not have any neurologic physical findings. The patient was noted to have decreased sensation in the oropharynx and larynx. He also had a CT of the neck and larynx, unremarkable.

PREOPERATIVE MEDICATION: Fentanyl 50 mcg IV, Versed 2 mg IV.

PROCEDURE: The Pentax video pediatric endoscope was passed with difficulty through the oropharynx. We could not get the patient to swallow properly, but we were able to get the scope down and there were no obstructing lesions. The gastroesophageal junction was seen at about 36 cm. Inspection of the esophagus revealed no erythema, ulceration, exudate, friability, or other mucosal abnormalities. From 36 to 38 cm was a 2-cm hiatal hernia. No lesions were seen in the hernia. The stomach proper was entered and the endoscope advanced to the second duodenum. Inspection in the second duodenum, first duodenum, duodenal bulb, and pylorus revealed no abnormalities. Retroflexion revealed no lesions in the cardia or lesser curvature. Inspection in the antrum, body, and fundus of the stomach revealed no abnormalities. The patient tolerated the procedure well.

IMPRESSION: Normal endoscopy, although difficult passage of the endoscope because of difficulty with patient's swallowing. There are no obstructing lesions present.

We then, with some difficulty, passed a ventral feeding tube and confirmed proper placement by auscultation; we will obtain x-rays before initiating tube feeding.

CPT Code(s): _____ 43235 _____

ICD-9-CM Code(s): _____ 793.4 _____ 787.20 _____

ICD-10-CM Code(s): _____ ✗ _____
                    Abn.find.GI   Dysphagia

Abstracting Questions

1. Would the diaphragmatic hernia be reported? _____ NO _____

Case 17: Colonoscopy with Biopsies

OPERATIVE REPORT

LOCATION: Outpatient, Hospital

PATIENT: Steve Barrett

PREOPERATIVE DIAGNOSIS: Hemoccult-positive stool.

POSTOPERATIVE DIAGNOSIS: Biopsies of two prominent folds in the rectal sigmoid region were cauterized and sampled, the potential being that these may be polyps, although this is not likely.

SURGEON: Daniel Olanka, MD

PREOPERATIVE MEDICATIONS: Demerol 50 mg IV; Versed 3 mg IV.

FINDINGS: The Pentax video colonoscope was inserted without difficulty to the cecum. The ileocecal valve was identified. The appendiceal orifice was seen. Careful inspection in the cecum, ascending colon, hepatic flexure, transverse colon, splenic flexure, descending colon, and sigmoid colon revealed no erythema, ulceration, exudate, friability, or other mucosal abnormalities. At the rectal sigmoid junction, there appeared to be a prominent fold versus polyp. This was gently cauterized and sampled. No other lesions were seen. The patient did have some internal hemorrhoids, not bleeding. The patient tolerated the procedure well.

IMPRESSION: Prominent fold versus polyp versus submucosal lesion biopsied and cauterized in the rectal sigmoid area. Internal hemorrhoids were not bleeding.

PLAN: The patient does not have a polyp; he should return for surveillance flexible sigmoidoscopy every 5 years and yearly rectals and hemoccults.

Pathology Report Later Indicated: Normal rectal tissue.

CPT Code(s): _45350_ (col w/ bio

ICD-9-CM Code(s): _792.1 m. x stool_ _455.0_

ICD-10-CM Code(s): _Contents_

Abstracting Questions

1. Was the source of the occult blood determined by the procedure? _no_
2. What is the primary diagnosis reported for the reason for the procedure? _blood in stool_

Chapter 3
Nephrology

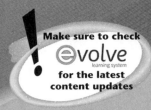

Make sure to check evolve learning system **for the latest content updates**

Case 18: Plasma Exchange

OPERATIVE REPORT

LOCATION: Outpatient, Hospital

PATIENT: Charles Jones

PROCEDURE PERFORMED: Plasmapheresis.

SURGEON: George Orbitz, MD

The patient was seen during plasmapheresis today for treatment of his myasthenia gravis. He has stable hemodynamics, no shortness of breath or dizziness. Exchange has been going well. We will continue to use the same 4-liter exchange replaced with 3 liters of 5% albumin mixed with calcium gluconate (3 amps) and potassium chloride (9 mEq), and with 1 liter of fresh frozen plasma. We will give him three exchanges and this is his final response.

CPT Code(s): _36514_

ICD-9-CM Code(s): _358.00_

ICD-10-CM Code(s): _____

Abstracting Questions

1. Would an E/M service also be reported? _____NO_____

2. Does the documentation indicate any exacerbation of the patient's condition? _____NO_____

3. Does the patient's "stable hemodynamics" status affect diagnosis coding? _____No_____

Therapeutic treatment

Case 19: Kidney Biopsy

OPERATIVE REPORT

LOCATION: Outpatient, Hospital

PATIENT: Lilly Brown

PREOPERATIVE DIAGNOSIS: Acute renal failure, possible rejection, possible ischemic nephropathy.

POSTOPERATIVE DIAGNOSIS: Same.

SURGEON: George Orbitz, MD

PROCEDURE PERFORMED: Transplant kidney biopsy.

PROCEDURE: The transplanted kidney in the right iliac fossa was visualized with ultrasound. The previous arteriovenous malformation was noted in the lower pole. We avoided that area as much as we could. At least three core biopsies were obtained after prepping the area in the usual fashion and injecting 1% lidocaine. A post-biopsy showed no evidence of hematoma or new AVM. The patient had some pain after the procedure and was sent to the post-procedure area. She will be getting some intravenous morphine.

Hemoglobin will be checked in 6 hours.

Pathology Report Later Indicated: Acute necrotizing glomerulitis.

CPT Code(s): _50200-RT, 76942_

ICD-9-CM Code(s): _580.4   V42.0 Post status (Already had transplant)_

ICD-10-CM Code(s): _____

Abstracting Questions

1. Was the biopsy done as an open procedure? _no_
2. What further reference is found when locating glomerulitis in the index? _nephritis_
3. What is AVM and is it reported? _Arterial venus malformation, no_

Case 20: Plasma Exchange

OPERATIVE REPORT

LOCATION: Outpatient, Hospital

PATIENT: Kindred Salsbury

PREOPERATIVE DIAGNOSIS: Myasthenia gravis.

POSTOPERATIVE DIAGNOSIS: Myasthenia gravis.

SURGEON: George Orbitz, MD

PROCEDURE PERFORMED: Plasma exchange #3.

PHYSICIAN: This patient underwent her third plasma exchange with a target volume of 3000. However, we replaced her with 5% albumin, cc for cc, and that totaled 3370, so the actual plasma removed was 4108 minus the 592 of ACDA, which resulted in 3516 cc of plasma, and this is fairly close. She did well. She had one transient drop in her pressure midway through and received saline. We gave her saline boluses three times, and she was stable, had no symptoms, and the entire procedure took 70 minutes today. Her pre and post vitals were stable. Her pre labs were reviewed and good, and the plan will include two more daily exchanges, a two-day interruption, a final exchange, and then a neurologic re-evaluation.

CPT Code(s): _____36514_____

ICD-9-CM Code(s): _____358.00_____

ICD-10-CM Code(s): _____

Abstracting Questions

1. Is the transient (temporary) drop in blood pressure reported? __no_____

Case 21: Kidney Biopsy

OPERATIVE REPORT

LOCATION: Outpatient, Hospital

PATIENT: Melissa Hart

SURGEON: George Orbitz, MD

PROCEDURE PERFORMED: Kidney biopsy.

REASON FOR PROCEDURE: Proteinuria. *Pre-op*

After the procedure and potential complications were explained to the patient and consent was obtained, she was prepped for a right native kidney biopsy. The area was prepped with Betadine solution. Sterile drapes were then applied around the area in the usual fashion. One-percent lidocaine was used as a local anesthetic, which was infiltrated in the intended biopsy site. The patient's right kidney was directly visualized prior to the procedure using ultrasound. After the lidocaine was given, a small skin incision was made at the biopsy site. The intended biopsy needle track was also infiltrated with lidocaine using a spinal needle under direct ultrasonographic guidance. A biopsy of the lower pole of the right kidney was taken with an 18-gauge Tru-Cut needle. Four attempts were made to obtain three good core samples. Postbiopsy ultrasound with color flow did not show any hematomas.

The patient tolerated the procedure well. There was minimal bleeding. There were no acute complications. She was given a total of 2 mg of Versed, with 100 mcg of Fentanyl for sedation and analgesia.

Pathology Report Later Indicated: Membranous glomerulonephritis. *Post-op*

CPT Code(s): _50200-Rt , 76942_

ICD-9-CM Code(s): _583.1_

ICD-10-CM Code(s): _____

Abstracting Questions

1. Was the biopsy of a transplanted kidney? _no_
2. Does this fact affect coding for the case? _no_
3. What type of glomerulonephritis is identified? _membranous_

Case 22: Central Venous Placement

OPERATIVE REPORT

LOCATION: Outpatient, Hospital

PATIENT: Harriet Smith

SURGEON: George Orbitz, MD

PROCEDURE PERFORMED: Tunneled triple-lumen central venous catheter.

ANESTHESIA: 1% lidocaine was used as a local anesthetic.

INDICATION: Intravascular access for dialysis because of acute renal failure.

PROCEDURE: After the procedure and its possible complications were explained and consent was obtained from the patient (age 46), she was prepped for left internal jugular tunneled triple-lumen catheter placement.

The area was sterilized using a standard Chloraprep solution. Sterile drapes were then applied around the area in the usual fashion. Under direct ultrasonographic guidance, an introducer needle was used to cannulate the patient's left internal jugular: Once in place, the J-tipped guidewire was inserted through the needle and advanced without any difficulty. The needle was subsequently removed. A small skin incision was made at the insertion site. A peel-away sheath with an internal dilator was then inserted over the guidewire using Seldinger technique. The guidewire was subsequently removed. The tunnel was created about 3 inches away from the internal jugular insertion site, below the left clavicle using a Hawkins needle. Once the tunnel was created, then the J-tipped guidewire was placed through the Hawkins needle. The Hawkins needle was subsequently removed. The preflushed 30-cm triple lumen Arrow catheter was then inserted through the tunnel over the guidewire. Once the catheter was through the tunnel, the guidewire was removed. The tip of the catheter was then inserted into the peel-away sheath up to the 23-cm mark. The peel-away sheath was then subsequently removed. The triple-lumen catheter was then secured into place using 2–0 sutures. Steri-Strips were then applied to the internal jugular insertion site.

The patient tolerated the procedure well. A subsequent chest x-ray showed that the tip of the catheter was well into the left atrium. The catheter was then subsequently withdrawn about 2 cm so that the tip was within the area of the superior vena cava.

There was minimal bleeding. There were no acute complications.

CPT Code(s): ___36558___   ___76942___

ICD-9-CM Code(s): ___584.9___

ICD-10-CM Code(s): _____

Abstracting Questions

1. Was this a tunneled catheter placement? ___yes___
2. Does the age of the patient affect the code selection? ___yes___
3. Does the insertion site of the catheter affect the CPT code selection? ___no___
4. What is the medical condition to be treated utilizing the central line? ___Acute renal failure___

Chapter 4
Neurology/Neurosurgery

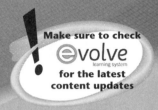

Case 23: Lumbar Puncture

OPERATIVE REPORT

LOCATION: Outpatient, Hospital

PATIENT: Susan Hildebrandt

PREOPERATIVE DIAGNOSIS: Intractable headache.

POSTOPERATIVE DIAGNOSIS: Same.

SURGEON: John Hodgson, MD

PROCEDURE PERFORMED: Lumbar puncture.

CONSENT: The risks and benefits were explained to the patient including pain, bleeding, headache, persistent CSF leak, and infection. She voiced understanding and signed the consent form.

DESCRIPTION: The patient was placed in the left lateral decubitus position. She was prepped and draped in a sterile fashion. One-percent lidocaine was infiltrated locally for anesthesia. A 22-gauge catheter was placed at the L4-5 interspace without difficulty. Approximately 12 cc of clear and slightly yellowish tinged fluid was removed. CSF was sent for analysis as ordered. Serum labs were also drawn to correlate with CSF. The patient tolerated this procedure well.

Pathology Report Later Indicated: Normal spinal fluid.

CPT Code(s): ___62270___

ICD-9-CM Code(s): ___784.0 Headache___

ICD-10-CM Code(s): _____

Abstracting Questions

1. How is this procedure listed in the index of the CPT? ___Spinal Tap___

2. Was this procedure diagnostic or therapeutic? _____

3. Is there a separate code available for *intractable* (unremitting, unrelenting, often non-responsive to usual treatment methods) headache? ___no___

Case 24: Electroencephalogram Report

LOCATION: Outpatient, Hospital

PATIENT: Judith Miller

PHYSICIAN: Timothy Pleasant, MD

Judith is a 53-year-old, right-handed female who had an EEG performed in the outpatient EEG lab. The EEG was performed on the 10-20 system with tin electrodes and collodion paste. No sedation was given. The time of last meal was 11:30 AM. This was non–sleep deprived. The EEG was performed in awake and drowsy states. Hyperventilation and photic stimulation were performed.

MEDICATIONS: Not listed.

INDICATION: Seizure prior to dialysis with history of lupus.

DESCRIPTION: Background rhythm is 10 to 11 cycles/second alpha, which is sometimes irregular. The waveforms do appear to be low amplitude, ranging from approximately 3 to 10 microvolts. There is intermittent beta activity noted. Waveforms occasionally become more in the 9-cycle/second area and will attenuate with eye opening during those brief moments. Hyperventilation of 3-minute duration good effort did not activate the effort. One to 25 Hz photic stimulation did not activate the record. There is a significant amount of muscle and movement artifact noted during the recording.

IMPRESSION: This is an abnormal EEG secondary to the low-voltage and occasional beta activity. Medications are not listed and could be seen in individuals with central nervous system activation such as benzodiazepines, barbiturates, or sometimes SSRIs. Clinical correlation is required.

CPT Code(s): _____ 95816   awake + drowsy EEG _____

ICD-9-CM Code(s): _____ 794.02   Abnormal, EEG _____ Seizure contributed to abnormal

ICD-10-CM Code(s): _____ 780.39 _____ reading

Abstracting Questions

1. What factors need to be considered when selecting a code for this EEG? _Awake, drowsy._

2. Does the lack of documentation of time affect the code selection? _no_

3. Did the EEG render a more specific seizure diagnosis? _no_

4. How would the "abnormal EEG" be reported in addition to seizures? _Abnormal or findings_

Case 25: Carpal Tunnel Release

OPERATIVE REPORT

LOCATION: Outpatient, Hospital

PATIENT: Henry Judge

PREOPERATIVE DIAGNOSIS: Left carpal tunnel syndrome.

POSTOPERATIVE DIAGNOSIS: Left carpal tunnel syndrome.

SURGEON: Johns Hodgson, MD

PROCEDURE PERFORMED: Left carpal tunnel release.

COMPLICATIONS: None.

INDICATION: This is a 58-year-old male with left carpal tunnel syndrome. He failed to respond to conservative treatment. After a discussion of the options and risks, he elected surgery.

PROCEDURE: The patient was taken to the operating room. He underwent IV sedation. The planned incision was infiltrated with local anesthetic and then an incision was made beginning at the base of the proximal phalanx in line between the 3rd and 4th metacarpals and extending to but not across the wrist crease. I cut the subcutaneous tissue and then sectioned the transverse carpal ligament. I initially exposed the median nerve and completed a proximal transection of the ligament and undermined the wrist crease. I then completed a distal transection of the ligament. The nerve was purplish colored. I was able to see more pink healthy-appearing nerve both at the proximal and distal ends of the decompression. I was content the nerve was adequately decompressed. I irrigated with copious amounts of saline. Subcutaneous tissue was closed with interrupted 2–0 Vicryl. The skin was closed with running 3–0 nylon stitches. A bulky dressing was placed. The patient tolerated the procedure well without apparent complications. Sponge, instrument, and needle counts were correct. He was moving his hand well after the surgery.

CPT Code(s): _____ 64721 – Lt _____

ICD-9-CM Code(s): _____ 354.0 _____

ICD-10-CM Code(s): _____

Abstracting Questions

1. Was this procedure open or through a scope? _____ open _____

2. Does the nerve involved affect the coding? _____ yes _____

3. What is a neuroplasty? _____ repair of the nerve _____

4. Where on the body is the "carpal tunnel"? _____ wrist _____

Case 26: Discectomy

OPERATIVE REPORT

LOCATION: Outpatient, Hospital

PATIENT: Neil Wills

PREOPERATIVE DIAGNOSIS: Left L5-S1 herniated disc.

POSTOPERATIVE DIAGNOSIS: Same.

SURGEON: John Hodgson, MD

PROCEDURE: Left L5-S1 discectomy.

INDICATIONS: This is a 37-year-old male who presented with left lower extremity pain. He had motor, sensory, and reflex findings all consistent with a left S1 radiculopathy. He had a large midline and, slightly to the left, a herniated L5-S1 disc. He failed to respond to conservative treatment. After discussion of the options and risks, he elected surgery.

PROCEDURE AS FOLLOWS: The patient was taken to the operating room and underwent induction of general endotracheal anesthesia in the supine position. He was then flipped over to the prone position on the operating room table. The lumbosacral area was sterilely prepped and draped. The C-arm was draped and moved into position. A K-wire was placed one fingerbreadth to the left of the L5-S1 interspace. This was confirmed with the C-arm. I then used a sequential series of dilators and eventually placed a 5-cm-long, 18-mm-diameter tubular retractor. This was verified again to be over the L5-S1 interspace with the C-arm. I then removed the redundant muscle with a Kerrison rongeur. I incised the ligamentum of flavum with a #15 blade and removed it with various sizes of Kerrison rongeurs. I retracted the common dural sac and the left S1 nerve root medially. There was a very significant bulge compressing the left S1 nerve root. I incised this and removed two large pieces of extruded disc. I then went into the disc space, which was narrow, and removed additional pieces of disc. At the end of the decompression, I could pass a nerve hook underneath the common dural sac across the midline, toward the right side, and I did not feel any further compression. I could also pass a nerve hook along the exiting S1 nerve root and did not feel any compression. At no time was there a dural tear or spinal fluid leak. I was content that the neural elements were nicely decompressed. I irrigated with copious amounts of saline. Surgicel was placed over the exposed dura. The tubular retractor was withdrawn. The subcutaneous tissue was closed with interrupted 2–0 Vicryl. The skin was closed with a running 3–0 Vicryl subcuticular stitch. Benzoin and ¼-inch Steri-Strips and a sterile dressing were placed. The patient tolerated the procedure well without apparent complications. Sponge, instrument, and needle counts were correct. He was taken to the recovery room in stable condition.

Pathology Report Later Indicated: Benign disc fragments.

CPT Code(s): _____ 63030 - Lt _____ Laminectomy _____

ICD-9-CM Code(s): _____ 722.10 Hern, displacement, lumbar _____

ICD-10-CM Code(s): _____

Abstracting Questions

1. When choosing the CPT code, is the location of the disc(s) a factor? _yes - lumbosacral area_

2. Does the number of discs involved affect code selection? _yes_

3. What is the direction when referencing the Index of the ICD-9-CM under the terms "Hernia, disc"?
   Displacement

Case 27: Ventricular Puncture

OPERATIVE REPORT

LOCATION: Outpatient, Hospital

PATIENT: Sam Dillard

PREOPERATIVE DIAGNOSIS: Increased intracerebral pressure.

POSTOPERATIVE DIAGNOSIS: Same.

SURGEON: John Hodgson, MD

OPERATIVE PROCEDURE: Percutaneous aspiration of ventricular reservoir.

Puncture

COMPLICATIONS: None.

INDICATIONS: This is a 19-year-old male with a high-grade glioma of the posterior fossa. He has shunt-dependent hydrocephalus due to the neoplasm. He comes to my office complaining of nausea, vomiting, lethargy, and headache. After obtaining consent from the parents, I went ahead and tapped the valve.

PROCEDURE: The patient was placed in the lateral supine position with the right side up. His neck and head was supported with a pillow. I prepped the site of the shunt reservoir with Betadine. I then took a 23-gauge needle attached to a 60-cc syringe and aspirated approximately 55 cc of xanthochromic CSF that had some particulate matter in it. I then withdrew the needle. I sent the fluid for total protein, glucose, cell count with differential, Gram stain culture, and Vancomycin level. The patient tolerated the procedure well. The needle was withdrawn. There were no complications.

Pathology Report Later Indicated: Normal cerebral spinal fluid.

CPT Code(s): _____ 61020 Vent, puncture _____

ICD-9-CM Code(s): _____ 191.6 Neo, cereb _____ 331.4 Hydro _____

ICD-10-CM Code(s): _____

Abstracting Questions

1. Does the route of entry for the needle affect the code selection? _____ Yes _____
2. Was there injection as well as aspiration? _____ no _____
3. What is the underlying condition? _____ High-grade glioma _____
4. Is there a second diagnosis to report? _____ Hydocephalus _____

Case 28: Electroencephalogram Report

LOCATION: Outpatient, Hospital

PATIENT: Henry Hartford

PHYSICIAN: Timothy Pleasant, MD

The patient was awake at the start of this EEG but was drowsy during a portion of the recording. This EEG was requested for evaluation of rapidly progressive dementia.

MEDICATIONS: Aricept, calcium, Colace, Fosamax, multivitamins, Flomax, and Benefiber.

The background activity was somewhat poorly organized, seemed rather diffuse, and consisted of 5 to 7 Hz theta activity, with amplitudes of 30 to 40 microvolts. Some beta activity was seen anteriorly. There was a partial alerting response to opening of the eyes.

The most significant feature of the recording was the frequent occurrence of paroxysmal bursts of 2 to 4 Hz delta and theta activity sometimes with amplitudes greater than 70 microvolts. These were most prominent anteriorly. Some sharply contoured waves were seen, especially in the left frontal area. These bursts of flow activity continued during drowsiness. Photic stimulation did not produce driving responses on either side.

IMPRESSION: This was an abnormal EEG because of:
1. Excessive slowing and disorganization of the background.
2. Paroxysmal bursts of delta activity, maximum anteriorly.

These findings indicate a generalized disturbance of cerebral function, which appears to be anterior. There are a few paroxysmal qualities, but no definite epileptiform activity was seen. These findings are compatible with various types of encephalopathies.

CPT Code(s): _____95816_____

ICD-9-CM Code(s): ___794.02   Abnormal EEG   294.8 Dementia___

ICD-10-CM Code(s): _____

Abstracting Questions

1. Would the diagnosis be reported as the presenting problem, or the results "abnormal EEG"? _Dementia_

Case 29: Insertion of Intrathecal Catheter and Pump

OPERATIVE REPORT

LOCATION: Outpatient, Hospital

PATIENT: Josh Ring

PREOPERATIVE DIAGNOSES
1. Osteoporosis.
2. Multiple compression fractures of the spine, status post multilevel kyphoplasty.
3. Lumbar spinal stenosis without neurogenic claudication.
4. Degenerative disc disease of the lumbar spine.
5. Alzheimer's disease.
6. Benign prostatic hypertrophy.

POSTOPERATIVE DIAGNOSES: Same.

SURGEON: John Hodgson, MD

PROCEDURE PERFORMED: Insertion of permanent intrathecal catheter and SynchroMed pump.

ANESTHESIA: General.

ESTIMATED BLOOD LOSS: Minimal.

PROCEDURE: The patient was brought to the operating room. General endotracheal anesthesia was instituted. He was placed in left lateral position. Parts were prepped and draped. Fluoroscopy guidance was obtained. Skin and subcutaneous tissue at the site of back incision, site of needle insertion, and right lower quadrant incision and tunneling tract were infiltrated with local anesthetic, 0.25% Sensorcaine with epinephrine; total amount used was 25 cc. I attempted to do the spinal tap at L5-S1, L4-L5 level under fluoroscopy guidance. I was unable to do that. I made the spinal tap at L3-4 level in one attempt without any difficulty. CSF was clear. There was free flow. Under fluoroscopy guidance, I inserted intraspinal catheter to T9 level. Stylet was removed. The flow was excellent. Under fluoroscopy guidance, I withdrew the intraspinal needle 1 cm making sure the intraspinal catheter did not get dislodged.

I made an incision, 3 inches long, in the right lower quadrant and carried that into the subcutaneous tissue. I made a pocket over abdominal wall fascia by blunt and sharp dissection. Hemostasis was achieved. This pocket was packed with antibiotic solution–soaked lap pad.

I made an incision in the back 2 inches long vertical along the intraspinal needle. I carried that incision into the subcutaneous tissue and made a pocket over the back muscle fascia by blunt and sharp dissection to accommodate the anchoring device. I placed 2–0 silk pursestring suture times two around the intraspinal needle. Intraspinal needle was removed under fluoroscopy guidance making sure the intraspinal catheter did not get dislodged. Pursestring sutures were tightened around the intraspinal catheter. This was done to prevent CSF leak around the intraspinal catheter. After tightening the pursestring sutures, I made sure the CSF flow was adequate through the catheter. Then I inserted anchoring device on the intraspinal catheter; the anchor was secured to back muscle fascia with 2–0 silk suture times two. I passed a tunneler from right lower quadrant incision into the back incision in one pass, then brought the intraspinal catheter through the right lower quadrant incision. Excess portion of the catheter was trimmed. Implanted catheter length is 64 cm with volume of 0.141 ml. Pump was made ready by the scrub nurse and Medtronics clinical specialist. It was filled with Bupivacaine and

Dilaudid solution. I connected the connecting tube to the intraspinal catheter. Connection was secured with 2–0 silk tie. This connection was connected to the pump, and this connection was secured with 0 silk tie.

Lap pad in the pump pocket was removed. Hemostasis was checked. Pump pocket was irrigated with antibiotic solution. The pump was placed in its pocket, making sure the filling port is anterior. The pump was secured to abdominal wall fascia with 0 silk suture at each anchoring site, one on the inferior side and one on the lateral side of the pump.

Both incisions were checked for hemostasis. They were irrigated with antibiotic solution. They were closed in two layers, 0 Vicryl interrupted for subcutaneous tissue, 3–0 Monocryl for subcuticular. Incisions were clean. Dermabond was applied. Pump was programmed to deliver Bupivacaine 5 mg and Dilaudid 500 mcg per day.

Pathology Report Later Indicated: Normal cerebral spinal fluid.

CPT Code(s): _62350_ cath _62362_ perp _77003_ fluid UHrasound

ICD-9-CM Code(s): _733.00_ , _724.02_ , _722.52_

ICD-10-CM Code(s): _Osteop_ , _Stenosis_ _Deg.disk_

Abstracting Questions

1. Was the catheterization of the spinal cord done during a laminectomy? _no_

2. Does the placement of the intrathecal catheter include insertion of the pump? _no_

3. Was the pump programmable? _yes_

4. Does this affect the code selection? _yes_

5. What are the primary diagnoses for the insertion of the pump? _Osteo, Lumbar stenosis_
   _#1   #3_

Chapter 5
Obstetric and Gynecologic Surgery and Ophthalmology

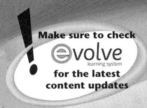

Make sure to check **evolve** learning system **for the latest content updates**

Case 30: Hysteroscopy

OPERATIVE REPORT

LOCATION: Outpatient, Hospital

PATIENT: Calley Olson

PREOPERATIVE DIAGNOSIS: Postmenopausal bleeding.

POSTOPERATIVE DIAGNOSIS: Endometrial polyp.

SURGEON: Andy Martinez, MD

OPERATIVE PROCEDURE: Diagnostic hysteroscopy with polypectomy and dilation and curettage.

PREAMBLE: The patient is a 42-year-old woman seen with complaints of postmenopausal bleeding. An attempt at endometrial biopsy in the office was, unfortunately, unsuccessful. The patient is therefore taken to the operating room for diagnostic hysteroscopy with D&C.

PROCEDURE NOTE: The patient was taken to the operating room and a general anesthetic was administered. The patient was then prepped and draped in the usual manner in the lithotomy position, and straight catheterization of the bladder was carried out. A weighted speculum was placed to allow for visualization of the cervix, which was grasped anteriorly using single-toothed tenaculum. The cervix was then dilated to allow for insertion of the diagnostic hysteroscope. Uterine cavity was entered, and there were two small endometrial polyps visible. Attempt was made to resect these with the hysteroscopic scissors, but unfortunately, this was unsuccessful. The hysteroscopic resecting loop, unfortunately, could not be made operational and could not be used.

Polyp forceps was therefore placed, and a small amount of the polypoid tissue was grasped for biopsy. A sharp curettage was also carried out with minimal products obtained.

The patient tolerated the procedure well and went to the recovery room in good condition. There were no complications. Estimated blood loss was minimal.

Pathology Report Later Indicated: Benign endometrial polyp.

CPT Code(s): ___58555___

ICD-9-CM Code(s): ___621.0___

ICD-10-CM Code(s): _____

Abstracting Questions

1. What was the route of approach for this procedure? __Vaginal_____

2. Was this procedure only diagnostic? __No_____

3. What definitive procedures were performed? __Biopsy, D+C_____

4. How many codes are required to report the diagnostic hysteroscopy, biopsy, and curettage? __1____

5. Is there a <u>definitive diagnosis</u> to report, or is the presenting problem reported? _____

Case 31: Amniocentesis

OPERATIVE REPORT

LOCATION: Outpatient, Hospital

PATIENT: Jennifer Barron

PREOPERATIVE DIAGNOSES
1. Intrauterine pregnancy at 32 plus weeks.
2. Insulin-dependent diabetes, type II.
3. Diabetic nephropathy. *250.40*

POSTOPERATIVE DIAGNOSIS: Same.

SURGEON: Andy Martinez, MD

PROCEDURE PERFORMED: Amniocentesis.

INDICATIONS: The patient is a 23-year-old with a complicated pregnancy who has been on bed rest because of diabetic nephropathy. Due to the fact that the fetus might be in a hostile environment, we believed that accelerated pulmonary maturity might be a possibility; therefore, at this time we elected to go with amniocentesis to help us manage her pregnancy. She had been fully informed of the risks and benefits of the procedure prior to proceeding.

DESCRIPTION OF PROCEDURE: The technologist did ultrasound scanning, and the placenta was posterior. We prepped the abdomen and draped it. We used a sterile covered ultrasound transducer with guide and located a pocket of fluid. The 20-gauge needle was inserted. As we got into the uterus the baby moved into the area, therefore the needle was immediately withdrawn; the fetus was palpated a little bit, and we stimulated the baby and it moved out of the area. We then repositioned the transducer and were able to drop into the pocket of amniotic fluid and withdrew 20 cc of clear yellow amniotic fluid. The fluid was sent for maturity studies. The patient tolerated the procedure without difficulty.

CPT Code(s): _____ *59000* _____ *76946 ~ Ultrasonic guide*

ICD-9-CM Code(s): _____ *250.40, 583.81, V58.67, 648.03* _____

ICD-10-CM Code(s): _____

Abstracting Questions

1. Is the procedure diagnostic or therapeutic? _____ *Diagnostic* _____

2. Is the ultrasound guidance included or <u>separately</u> reported? _____

3. Does the pregnancy affect the primary diagnosis code selection? _____ *yes complicated*

4. What is the fifth digit classification for this patient? _____ *0* _____

5. Would the diabetes and nephropathy also be reported? _____ *yes* _____

6. Is the diabetic code selection influenced by the nephropathy? _____ *yes* _____

Case 32: Dacryocystorhinostomy

OPERATIVE REPORT

LOCATION: Outpatient, Hospital

PATIENT: Hilldy Johannasen

PREOPERATIVE DIAGNOSES
1. Chronic dacryocystitis, left.
2. Hypertension.
3. Status post cataract surgery, right eye.
4. Glaucoma, chronic open angle, both eyes.
5. Benign meningioma.
6. Type II diabetes.
7. Hypothyroidism.
8. Cellulitis secondary to #1.

POSTOPERATIVE DIAGNOSES
1. Chronic dacryocystitis, left.
2. Hypertension.
3. Status post cataract surgery, right eye.
4. Glaucoma, chronic open angle, both eyes.
5. Benign meningioma.
6. Type II diabetes.
7. Hypothyroidism.
8. Cellulitis secondary to #1.

SURGEON: Rita Wimer, MD

68720

PROCEDURE PERFORMED: Left dacryocystorhinostomy with left canalicular intubation with silicone.

ANESTHESIA: General endotracheal anesthesia.

INDICATION: This 78-year-old white female has had chronic cellulitis and pus discharge from her left eye for the last 2 or 3 years, which has just progressively gotten worse to where she now has almost a fistula between the lacrimal sac and the skin. The chronic infection is draining her financially and taking its sap on her general health. She was counseled as to the type of repair, risk for infection, anesthesia, presence of a tube, and postoperative care.

DESCRIPTION OF PROCEDURE: After the patient had been given Cleocin 900 mg IV in the holding area, she was prepped and draped in the usual sterile fashion for ophthalmic surgery under general anesthesia. The lateral and medial canthi were marked, as were the connecting lines between the canthi. Ten millimeters from the left medial canthus an 11-mm incision was marked with a sterile marking pen. A #15 Bard-Parker blade was used to cut down to the periosteum, and the insulated Bovie tip was used. The Freer periosteal elevator was used to free up the periosteum over the anterior lacrimal crest, and the nose was entered with a freer elevator. The Kerrison small, middle, and large rongeurs were used to create a 14-mm bony osteotomy. Copious pus was coming from the lacrimal sac and through the canalicular system superiorly. This was cultured and sent to the lab. A #12 Bard-Parker blade was then used to take off the posterior medial walls. This was found to be thickened, and again more pus was removed, but no stones. The nasal sinus mucosa was also removed and sent to the lab along with the bony osteotomy specimens and the lacrimal wall specimens. The Guibor tube was then passed through the superior and inferior system after a punctum dilator was used. This was brought out through the common canaliculus and pulled out through the nose. 3–0 silk ties, two in the osteotomy and one distally, were then used to tie the tube. A Bacitracin-soaked glove was then passed along the tube into the wound and sutured with 6–0 nylon at the tip of the nose. The Guibor tube was cut and allowed to retract into the nose. The wound was closed with a running subcuticular 6–0 black nylon with three interrupted black nylons. Steri-Strips were used. Maxitrol ointment, Telfa pad, and patch were applied. The patient was sent to the recovery room. A mustache dressing was used. Estimated blood loss was less than 50 cc. There were no complications.

Pathology Report Later Indicated: Normal culture.

CPT Code(s): _____68720_____

ICD-9-CM Code(s): _____375.42_____

ICD-10-CM Code(s): _____

Abstracting Questions

1. Was the procedure done with an open approach or via endoscope? ___open___

2. Does the chronic status affect diagnosis code selection? ___yes___

3. Are other preoperative conditions reported for this procedure? ___no___

Case 33: Blepharoplasty

OPERATIVE REPORT

LOCATION: Outpatient, Hospital

PATIENT: Anna Penn

PREOPERATIVE DIAGNOSES
1. Upper lid entropion, each eye.
2. History of herpes simplex keratitis, left eye.
3. Diabetes mellitus type I.

POSTOPERATIVE DIAGNOSES: Same.

SURGEON: Rita Wimer, MD

PROCEDURE: Wedge resection with mini-blepharoplasty, upper lids, OU (both eyes).

ANESTHESIA: MAC (Monitored Anesthesia Care).

INDICATION: This 45-year-old white female has had recurrent eye pain and irritation of her eye secondary to upper lid entropion, both eyes. She was counseled as to the repair, risk for infection, recurrence, and exposure.

DESCRIPTION OF PROCEDURE: After the patient was prepped and draped in the usual sterile fashion for ophthalmic surgery, the amount of skin to be resected was determined by the open eye/close eye method. This was marked with a sterile marking pen and infiltrated with 2% Xylocaine with 0.75% Marcaine and bicarbonate. A #15 Bard-Parker blade then made a free hand dissection, and a 2-mm strip of orbicularis was removed. Epinephrine soaked sponges were then applied for 10 minutes under cool water compresses, and the cautery was used. It was determined that no fat was prolapsing and that the fat pads were left undisturbed. The wound was then closed with multiple interrupted 6–0 nylon sutures, and Maxitrol ointment, Telfa, and two half-eye pads were applied. There were no complications.

Pathology Report Later Indicated: Benign tissue.

CPT Code(s): ~~15622~~ 67923-50 (Repair) Eyelids

ICD-9-CM Code(s): 374.00

ICD-10-CM Code(s): _____

Abstracting Questions

1. Does the wedge resection method affect code selection? _____ yes

2. How is the bilateral treatment reported? _____ -50

3. Does the unspecified type of entropion affect diagnosis code selection? _____ no

4. Does the diabetes need to be reported? _____ no

Case 34: Removal Caruncle

OPERATIVE REPORT

LOCATION: Outpatient, Hospital

PATIENT: Celine Ripple

PREOPERATIVE DIAGNOSIS: Pigmented lesion, <u>caruncle</u>, of right eye.

POSTOPERATIVE DIAGNOSIS: Same.

SURGEON: Rita Wimer, MD

PROCEDURE PERFORMED: Removal of caruncle, right eye.

ANESTHESIA: General endotracheal anesthesia.

INDICATION: This 64-year-old white female has had a progressively enlarging pigmented lesion on the right conjunctiva. This has enlarged dramatically and she is very frightened that it could be malignant. It does have ragged edges and stays right on the conjunctiva. She was counseled for the procedure and because of her hyperanxiety it was done under general.

PROCEDURE: After she was prepped and draped in the usual sterile fashion under general anesthesia, the wire lid speculum was used to separate the lids of the right eye. The caruncle, measuring 0.6 cm, was found to be isolated and the pigmented lesion occupied almost the entire inferior half. Grasping this gently with the tissue forceps, this was carefully dissected away with a #69 Beaver blade. The lesion was sent intact to the pathology department, and the entire caruncle was removed. Wet-field cautery was used and then 2 minutes of application of epinephrine soaked sponges for one minute by the clock. It was elected not to do suturing since there would appear to be a cicatrix (scar) created, and the conjunctiva was allowed to flap over the site of the old caruncle and there was full extraocular motility. TobraDex ointment, Telfa, and two eye pads were applied, and the patient was sent to the recovery area. There were no complications.

Pathology Report Later Indicated: Benign tissue.

CPT Code(s): _____ 68110-Rt _____ Excision _____

ICD-9-CM Code(s): _____ 372.00 _____

ICD-10-CM Code(s): _____

Abstracting Questions

1. What is the location of the caruncle (lesion, fleshy outgrowth)? _Rt eye_
2. Does the size of the caruncle affect the CPT selection? _yes_
3. Does the location of the caruncle affect ICD-9-CM selection? _yes_

Chapter 6
Orthopedic

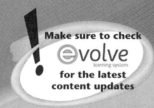

Case 35: Anterior Cruciate Ligament Reconstruction

OPERATIVE REPORT

LOCATION: Outpatient, Hospital

PATIENT: Morris Valley

PREOPERATIVE DIAGNOSIS: Status post right knee meniscal repair now secondary staged *Derangement* anterior cruciate ligament reconstruction.

POSTOPERATIVE DIAGNOSIS: Anterior cruciate ligament deficit, right knee. *Tear*

SURGEON: Mohomad Almaz, MD

PROCEDURE PERFORMED: Anterior cruciate ligament reconstruction.

ANESTHESIA: General.

PROCEDURE: After satisfactory level of general anesthesia, the patient was placed in a supine position and the extremity was prepped and draped in routine sterile manner. Exam at this time under anesthesia showed that he has continuation of a grade 2+ ACL deficiency positive pivot shift.

Upon entering the joint through routine established arthroscopic portals, it was significant to note the suprapatellar pouch was unremarkable. Patella had areas of grade 1 osteoarthritic change similar to the type of changes of grade 1 to 2 varieties about the intercondylar notch.

Medial gutter was unremarkable. Medial compartment was significant for documented and demonstrated excellent repair and healing of the medial meniscus. The articular surface had scant areas of diffuse grade 1 osteoarthritic change. The notch proper at this time was addressed, completing a more formal definitive notch plasty, and with completion of this the lateral compartment was well visualized and unremarkable in its appearance. The articular surfaces and the meniscus were pristine in their character.

Through the arthroscopic portals, I simply proceeded at this time with the advancement of a guide pin and simultaneous to this we also created an anterior-based incision sharply dissecting down to the prepatellar fascia. The fascia was then further incised. Also, at this interval in time, we proceeded with harvesting of the central $\frac{1}{3}$ of the patellar tendon with use of bone-tendon-bone construct of 10 mm in width, 25 mm in length from both the tibia and the tibial tubercle. This was then further prepared on the back table. The prior placed tibial guide pin was in excellent position in the remnant stump of the ACL. I then simply proceeded to over-ream about the guide pin, creating a 10-mm channel. This was then further followed by advancement of a Beeth needle in the 11-o'clock position. The needle was advanced, and over advanced needle use of acorn reamer created a 40-mm × 10-mm channel within the femoral advanced.

The Beeth needle was then used to advance the prior prepared reconstruction ACL graft. The advancement of this within the femoral tunnel and with use of counter distraction, a guide pin, was placed through guide pin. A bioabsorbable screw was used to fixate the femoral elements of the graft. This was then further followed by advancement of a bioabsorbable interference screw about the tibial tunnel in the graft. At this setting, the knee was without encumbrance to movement other than that limited by the table at approximately 115 degrees of flexion. At this time there was no demonstration as to positive Lachman's test findings and/or pivot shift through limited arcs of movement as above. There was no abutment, as noted arthroscopically.

After completion of this element of the procedure, the knee was evacuated of irrigating material, donor site closed in an interrupted manner, followed by whipstitch closure of the fascia. Portal sites were also closed. Indwelling Stryker pain pump was placed.

Estimated blood loss was minimal. Tourniquet time for the procedure was 62 minutes. Sponge and needle counts were correct. There were no noted complicating events. The patient tolerated the procedure well. Intraoperative photos were obtained as well for documentation.

CPT Code(s): _____29666-RT_____

ICD-9-CM Code(s): ____717.83_____

ICD-10-CM Code(s): _____

Abstracting Questions

1. Was the procedure open or <u>arthroscopic</u>? _____

2. Does the specific ligament repaired affect code selection? __yes_____

3. Is the harvest of the tendon graft reported separately? ____no_____

Case 36: Meniscectomy

OPERATIVE REPORT

LOCATION: Outpatient, Hospital

PATIENT: Conrad Hope

PREOPERATIVE DIAGNOSIS: Internal derangement of right knee.

POSTOPERATIVE DIAGNOSES
1. Grade III osteoarthritis lateral femoral condyle.
2. Grade II osteoarthritis medial tibial plateau.
3. Grade II osteoarthritis lateral tibial plateau.
4. Grade I/II osteoarthritis medial femoral condyle.
5. Grade II/III osteoarthritis medial facet of patella.

[handwritten: Tear – medial 836.0 lateral 836.1   osteo – lower leg]

SURGEON: Mohomad Almaz, MD

PROCEDURE PERFORMED
1. Partial medial and lateral meniscectomies. *[handwritten: 29880]*
2. Excision of plica.
3. Limited abrasion chondroplasty lateral femoral condyle.
4. Noted anterior cruciate ligament–deficient knee.

PROCEDURE: After a satisfactory level of general anesthesia with the patient in the supine position, the extremity was prepped and draped in a routine sterile manner. Establishment of arthroscopic portals then further followed this. Upon entering the right knee, the patella and its tracking were unremarkable other than the arthritic changes of the fat pad, which abutted the most and is noted above. There was also a large redundant medial margin of the medial femoral condyle.

For the sake of visualization, the fat pad was excised at this time with plical entity, and the cartilage surfaces of the patella underwent abrasion chondroplasty.

Also at this time, the medial meniscus was well identified. There was a posterior medial meniscal tear. This was requiring of a debridement and trimming back to stable margin. There were some areas of diffuse arthritic change about the articular surfaces, as noted above, but were not addressed with mechanical end-cutting device. The articular notch was negative with the exception of ACL noted deficiency, as well as the demonstration of metastasis of the ACL to the PCL.

Lateral compartment was well visualized. Further at this time, this did demonstrate that there was a tearing of the posterior horn and the circumferential mid one-third of the lateral meniscus. At this time this was trimmed back to stable margin. Articular surfaces were then addressed, given areas of arthritic change, as noted above, with abrasion chondroplasty of lateral femoral condyle. At the completion of this element of the procedure, portal sites were closed followed by therapeutic injection of 5 cc of 1% Marcaine with 1 cc of Depo-Medrol 80 mg/cc, further followed by application of sterile dressings. The patient was transferred to the recovery room in a stable manner.

CPT Code(s): _____ *[handwritten: 29880–Rt   29877–Rt]*

ICD-9-CM Code(s): _____ *[handwritten: 836.0   836.1   715.96]*

ICD-10-CM Code(s): _____

Abstracting Questions

1. Is the partial meniscectomy coded as excision or _repair?_ _____

2. Is coding affected by if one or both menisci are treated? _yes_ _____

3. Is the patellar abrasion reported separately? _no_ _____

4. Are each of the meniscal tear diagnosis codes reported? _yes_ _____

5. Is the plical entity of the fat pad diagnosis reported? _no_ _____

6. What diagnosis would provide medical necessity for the abrasion chondroplasty? _osteoarthritis_

Case 37: Synovectomy

OPERATIVE REPORT

LOCATION: Outpatient, Hospital

PATIENT: Theodore Schumer

PREOPERATIVE DIAGNOSES
1. Left knee medial femoral condyle fracture.
2. Retained metal, left knee.

Complication – mech, device nonabsorbable surgical material

POSTOPERATIVE DIAGNOSES: Same.

SURGEON: Mohomad Almaz, MD

PROCEDURE PERFORMED: Left knee arthroscopy with synovectomy and metal removal and manipulation under general anesthesia. *29874 29877 Lt*

| Removal of staple

ANESTHESIA: General.

ESTIMATED BLOOD LOSS: Minimal.

DRAINS: None.

PROCEDURE: A 28-year-old male 6 weeks status post medial femoral condyle fracture on the left. He underwent open reduction internal fixation. He was taken back to surgery. After appropriate level of anesthesia was achieved, the left knee was appropriately prepped and draped in orthopedic manner. We made two portals in the knee, one medial and the other lateral to the patellar tendon. Sharp dissection was carried through the skin and blunt dissection was carried into the joint space. On examination of the knee we appreciated that the patient had extensive scarring in the suprapatellar area and the medial gutter. This was debrided with a shaver. We appreciated some scarring in the femoral notch area but this was debrided. The patient had a nonfunctioning anterior cruciate ligament tear. The medial and lateral meniscus were probed and felt to be intact. The fracture site was identified. We could appreciate no gross motion with palpation or range of motion across the fracture site.

We manipulated the knee but we could not get more than 45 degrees of flexion. For fear of suffering a fracture or rupture, we did not do any further aggressive manipulation. There was appreciated a metal staple in the femoral notch area. This appeared to be loose. We went ahead and pulled it out through the scope. We repaired the portal sites with interrupted nylon sutures and dressed the wound sterilely. The patient was placed in an Ace wrap. The patient appeared to tolerate the procedure well and left the operating room in good condition.

CPT Code(s): _____ *29874, 29877* _____

ICD-9-CM Code(s): _____ *996.59* _____

ICD-10-CM Code(s): _____

Abstracting Questions

1. Is the synovium actually excised? _____ *Yes* _____

2. Is removal of the retained loose staple reported? _____ *Yes* _____

3. How is the diagnosis for the removal of the staple located in the Index? _____ *Complication* _____

Case 38: Closed Reduction

OPERATIVE REPORT

LOCATION: Outpatient, Hospital

PATIENT: Patrick Jutes

PREOPERATIVE DIAGNOSIS: Displaced intra-articular distal left radius fracture. *perc. fixation* [handwritten: 2 1 3]

POSTOPERATIVE DIAGNOSIS: Same.

SURGEON: Mohomad Almaz, MD

PROCEDURE PERFORMED: Closed reduction and external fixator application, distal left radius fracture. *[handwritten: Fracture, radius, lower, toward wrist]*

ANESTHESIA: General anesthesia.

PROCEDURE: The patient was brought to the operating room, and general anesthetic was induced. The left upper extremity was hung in finger-trap traction with 5 pounds of counterweight. We then exsanguinated the limb, and tourniquet was inflated to 250 mm Hg for 35 minutes. We manipulated the distal radius fracture and used the C-arm in AP (anterior/posterior views) and lateral planes to confirm excellent reduction of the articular surface and restitution of length of the distal radius. We therefore prepped the arm with Betadine and draped it in a sterile fashion. We proceeded with application of an external fixator, applying two pins into the base of the index metacarpal and two pins in the radial shaft more proximally and connected these with stacked external carbon fiber bars. The appearance of the pins and reduction of the fracture was excellent on the C-arm views. We cut off excess pin length. We then applied Xeroform about the pins and applied a compression long-arm Robert–Jones dressing with plantar splints immobilizing the arm at 90-degree flexion. The patient tolerated the procedure well. The tourniquet was released prior to this, and good circulation returned to the arm. He went to the recovery room in excellent condition. He will be dismissed as an outpatient today with plans for follow-up back in the office in two weeks. Discharge medication included Lorcet, 30 tablets.

CPT Code(s): _____ *25606-LT* _____

ICD-9-CM Code(s): _____ *813.42* _____

ICD-10-CM Code(s): _____

Abstracting Questions

1. Which would be reported, the closed reduction or the external fixation? _____

2. Is the fracture open or closed? _____

3. Does the specific bone involved affect the diagnosis code? _____ *yes* _____

4. What else affects the diagnosis code? _____ *Location* _____

Case 39: Arthroplasty

OPERATIVE REPORT

LOCATION: Outpatient, Hospital

PATIENT: Milly Hutton

PREOPERATIVE DIAGNOSIS: Painful nonunion, right fifth toe distal phalanx.

POSTOPERATIVE DIAGNOSIS: Same.

SURGEON: Mohomad Almaz, MD

PROCEDURE PERFORMED: Excision of nonunion bone fragment distal phalanx, right fifth toe arthroplasty.

ANESTHESIA: Local sedation. Approximately 3 cc of a 50/50 mixture of 1% lidocaine plain and 0.5% Marcaine plain.

HEMOSTASIS: Ankle cuff, 250 mm of Mercury on the right for approximately 16 minutes.

ESTIMATED BLOOD LOSS: Minimal

COMPLICATIONS: None

SUTURES UTILIZED: 3–0 undyed Vicryl, 4–0 undyed Vicryl, 5–0 nylon

INJECTABLES POSTOPERATIVE: 1 cc of dexamethasone.

CLINICAL RESUME: This is a 30-year-old who presents approximately 6 months following injury to right fifth toe. The patient was evaluated initially with this. X-rays were done. X-rays were really inconclusive at the time for any kind of fracture. She continued to have pain and swelling to the toe. Repeat x-rays were done that indicated a fracture at the distal interphalangeal joint. Actually the patient has a congenital fusion of the distal interphalangeal joint. She only had one joint in the right fifth toe and I think what happened is this broke through the congenital fusion site and that is one of the reasons it did not heal, but she is continuing to be bothered with pain. We have tried splinting her, taping the toe, surgical shoe, and the x-rays indicate that it is just not healing, so the proposed surgery is mainly just to excise the fragment rather than try to repair it or get it to heal. It is too small of a bone. She does understand the proposed surgery risks and complications. I do not believe there is any infection. When I got in there today I could not see any signs of infection, it just looked like a nonunion or fibrous union. Part of it was healing, but the lateral aspect was soft and fibrous, kind of scar tissue. Otherwise everything appeared to be normal.

DESCRIPTION OF OPERATION: The patient was brought to the operating room and placed on the operating room table in the supine position. Administered IV sedation. Locally anesthetized about the right fifth toe. The right foot and leg were prepped and draped. Esmarch bandage applied from the tips of the toes to the ankle region. Ankle cuff was inflated to 250 mm of Mercury. Attention directed to the right fifth toe. Linear incision about 1 cm in length was made extending from the distal toe to the proximal phalanx, linear. Incision was deepened in the same surgical plane down to tendinous structures. Dissection was then carried bluntly along the medial and lateral aspect of the proximal and middle phalanx areas. Transverse tenotomy was done at the level of the proximal interphalangeal joint. Tendon was dissected off of the middle phalanx and trying to preserve the distal attachment. The Freer elevator was then utilized to find the fracture site; it was soft on the lateral aspect. The medial part did seem to be partially fused. There was some swelling around it, but I did utilize a #15 blade to cut through the nonunion site and then an oscillating saw to get the medial aspect. The bone was resected. The wound was flushed copiously with normal sterile saline. Bone otherwise did appear to be fairly normal. No osseous abnormalities, no other injuries noted. The extensor tendon was then reapproximated, as well as capsular structures with 3–0 Vicryl in simple interrupted fashion. Superficial fascial structures reapproximated with 4–0 Vicryl in simple interrupted fashion. The skin was closed with 5–0 nylon in simple interrupted fashion. Dexamethasone was infiltrated deep to the wound, about a cc was infiltrated. Adaptic, 4 × 4s, Kling, Kerlix, and Ace wrap were utilized for dressing material. Ankle cuff was deflated and normal vascular status did return to all digits of the right foot. The patient tolerated the procedure and anesthesia. The patient was discharged from the operating room to the same-day area with vital signs stable in apparent good condition.

CPT Code(s): _____26124 – 29_____

ICD-9-CM Code(s): _____733.82_____

ICD-10-CM Code(s): _____

Abstracting Questions

1. Was a portion of bone excised? _____yes_____

2. Is the tenotomy also reported? _____no_____

3. Is there a code for nonunion of the toe? _____yes_____

4. Would the anomaly of the toe be reported? _____yes_____ – 29 _____

Case 40: Mosaicplasty

OPERATIVE REPORT

LOCATION: Outpatient, Hospital

PATIENT: Jason Black

PREOPERATIVE DIAGNOSES
1. Internal derangement of right knee.
2. Known area of grade 4 arthritic change of the medial femoral condyle.

POSTOPERATIVE DIAGNOSES: Same.

SURGEON: Mohomad Almaz, MD

Arthroscopy, Knee

PROCEDURE PERFORMED: Mosaicplasty.

PROCEDURE: At this time in this regard under sterile technique, the patient underwent establishment of routine arthroscopic portals about the knee. Upon entering the knee proper, the patella and its tracking were only significant in that there were some scanty areas of grade 2 arthritic change with subtle fissuring of the mid cistern of the patella. The articular notch was otherwise unremarkable. There was some remnant of a plical type entity, which was trimmed back at this time for the sake of visualization. At this setting there was a focal area of approximately 1 cm^2 about the medial femoral condyle, which had a loose redundant flap-type tear and some overlaying very frail fibrous-type tissue. At this time in this regard the meniscus was propalpated and otherwise unremarkable. There was no reciprocating wear about the medial tibial plateau other than some scant areas of grade 1 arthritic change. The intra-articular notch had an A-frame–type notch. Cruciate structures were otherwise unremarkable. In the lateral compartment, the meniscus was propalpated and unremarkable other than some scant fraying about the circumferential inner one-third, but this is nonpathologic. He also had frank fissuring of grade 2/3 qualities about the medial tibial plateau, but this was without abnormal excursion or redundancy and required no definitive other management. At this time in this regard, I had some difficulties in trying to inflate the patella through a very limited mini-arthrotomy procedure. We simply proceeded with the harvesting of one 6.5-mm graft. The graft was then further prepared on the back table, and at this time we debrided the margins of the defect, medial and femoral condyle followed by drilling, dilating, and implanting arthroscopically the graft. This restored the contour and profile of the articular surfaces. It was confirmed arthroscopically. There was some light debris from the shavings, which was also removed at this time, and with propalpation demonstrated that the defect of the condyle was restored to approximately 90% of its full weight-bearing surface being covered with articular cartilage. The minimal areas of exposed bleeding bone were basically a non–weight-bearing entity. I filled the defects in an excellent manner and created no eburnate type of abutment throughout its course of range of movement. On completion of this, portal sites were simply closed. Limited mini-arthrotomy portal site was closed. The patient was transported to the recovery room in a stable manner.

CPT Code(s): _29866_

ICD-9-CM Code(s): _716.96_

ICD-10-CM Code(s): _____

Abstracting Questions

1. Is this an open or closed procedure? _____

2. Is the harvesting of the autograft included? __yes_____

Case 41: Arthroscopy

Assign an E code to indicate how the injury occurred.

OPERATIVE REPORT

LOCATION: Outpatient, Hospital

PATIENT: Kristine Millermann

PREOPERATIVE DIAGNOSIS: Right shoulder possible biceps tendon injury, possible labral injury, possible rotator cuff tear.

POSTOPERATIVE DIAGNOSIS: Right shoulder biceps tendon tear.

SURGEON: Mohomad Almaz, MD

PROCEDURES PERFORMED
1. Right shoulder arthroscopy. 29805-Rt
2. Open right biceps tenodesis. 23430 Reconstruction

CLINICAL HISTORY: This 26-year-old lady presents with a history of a right shoulder impingement type syndrome from several years ago. This had been operated on with an arthroscopy and had done well. About 2 months ago she began having increasing pain after sustaining a popping sensation within the shoulder. She had pain with continued supination. Biceps tests preoperatively were positive. An arthrogram was negative. After the risks and benefits of anesthesia and surgery were explained to the patient, a decision was made to undertake this procedure.

ANESTHESIA: Regional.

PROCEDURE: Under regional anesthetic, the patient was laid in the beach chair position on the operating table. The right shoulder was prepped and draped in usual fashion. The patient was given 1 gram of Cefazolin intravenously prior to surgery. A standard posterior arthroscopic portal was created and the camera introduced to the back of the joint. We had excellent visualization. An anterior portal was created using a switching stick technique, and the 7-mm cannula was then brought in from the front along with a blunt probe. Inspection of the articular surfaces showed no damage on the humerus or glenoid surfaces. There was some minor fraying of the anterior glenoid labrum. The biceps tendon was inspected and was found to have tearing through approximately 50% of the fiber structure. The biceps was then brought into the joint with the use of the probe and we could see that this extended through an area of approximately 2 cm. It was believed that this was the fundamental pathology. The rotator cuff was inspected. No further abnormalities could be identified on the humeral surface. The subacromial space was then entered through the posterior portal, and we could not see any damage to the rotator cuff on this surface.

Instruments were then removed from the joint. A lateral incision approximately 4 cm in length was made centered over the anterior aspect of the greater tuberosity. It was deepened through subcutaneous tissue to expose the deltoid fascia, which was then incised longitudinally and the deltoid bluntly split to expose the area of the bicipital groove. The biceps tendon was easily identified. The biceps tendon was then isolated and a suture was passed through it to hold its position. An arthroscopy camera was then placed into the posterior portal. The anterior portal was once again opened and the biceps was then transected using a scissors just near its attachment on the superior glenoid. The biceps was then brought in to the open wound laterally.

A drill hole was then made in the groove and two smaller drill holes proximally. A series of #5 Ethibond sutures were then woven through the biceps tendon. The four strands of suture were then brought in to the larger central hole and then two out on each side. The sutures were then tied onto themselves, pulling the biceps tendon into the large central hole to hold its position.

Once this was completed, the wound was irrigated with normal saline. The deltoid fascia was then repaired with 3–0 Vicryl suture. The skin was closed with Monocryl suture, and then the wound was dressed with Steri-Strips.

The wounds were then dressed with Mepore dressing and the arm placed in a Cryocuff sling. The patient was then awakened and placed on her hospital bed and taken to the recovery room in good condition. Estimated blood loss for the procedure was negligible. Sponge and needle counts were correct.

CPT Code(s): _____ 29805-Rt   23430-Rt _____

ICD-9-CM Code(s): _____ 840.6   E928.9 _____

ICD-10-CM Code(s): _____

Abstracting Questions

1. Should the diagnostic arthroscopy be reported in this case? _____ Yes _____

2. Is the tendon repair done with the scope or open? _____

3. Where does ICD-9-CM refer the biceps tendon tear to be reported? _____ sprain _____

Inj. Injured, nonspec. or nonclass   — Fade

Look-up

Chapter 7
Otorhinolaryngology

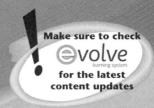

Make sure to check
evolve
learning system
**for the latest
content updates**

Case 42: Tympanostomy

OPERATIVE REPORT

LOCATION: Outpatient, Hospital

PATIENT: Shannon Johnson

PREOPERATIVE DIAGNOSIS: Chronic otitis media with effusion.

POSTOPERATIVE DIAGNOSIS: Same.

PROCEDURE PERFORMED: Bilateral tympanostomies with placement of ventilation tubes.

SURGEON: Jeff King, MD

FINDINGS: The patient had thick mucoid fluid behind both drums.

PROCEDURE: After the patient was placed under general anesthesia, the right canal was cleared of wax and prepped with Betadine. A radial incision was made in the anterior-inferior quadrant, and thick mucoid fluid was suctioned from behind this drum. A 0.39-mm ventilation tube was inserted. The left canal was then cleared of wax and prepped with Betadine. A radial incision was made in the anterior-inferior quadrant, and thick mucoid fluid was suctioned from behind this drum. A 0.39-mm ventilation tube was inserted. The canal was then filled with Ciprodex on both sides and cotton in the external auditory meatus. The patient was awakened from her anesthetic and returned to the recovery room in stable condition. Prognosis immediate/remote is good. Blood loss is 0.

CPT Code(s): _____ 69436-50 _____

ICD-9-CM Code(s): _____ 381.3 _____

ICD-10-CM Code(s): _____

Abstracting Questions

1. Does the insertion of the ventilating tube affect code selection? _yes   no_

2. Does the type of anesthesia affect the code selection? _yes_

3. Does the chronic status of the condition affect code selection? _yes_

4. Does the effusion status affect the code choice? _yes_

Case 43: Uvulopalatopharyngoplasty and Tonsillectomy

OPERATIVE REPORT

LOCATION: Outpatient, Hospital

PATIENT: Keith Hampton

PREOPERATIVE DIAGNOSES   *327.23*
1. Obstructive sleep apnea.
2. Recurrent tonsillitis.   *474.00*
3. Hypertrophic tonsils.
4. Hypertrophic uvula and palate.   *528.9*

POSTOPERATIVE DIAGNOSES
1. Obstructive sleep apnea.
2. Recurrent tonsillitis.
3. Hypertrophic tonsils.
4. Hypertrophic uvula and palate.

SURGEON: Jeff King, MD

PROCEDURES PERFORMED: 1. Uvulopalatopharyngoplasty. 2. Tonsillectomy.

ANESTHESIA: General endotracheal anesthesia.

INDICATION: A 32-year-old male with a history of recurrent tonsillitis. He also has obstructive sleep apnea. The patient is in for surgical treatment.

DESCRIPTION OF PROCEDURE: After consent was obtained, the patient was taken to the operating room and placed on the operating table in a supine position. After an adequate level of general endotracheal anesthesia was obtained, the patient was turned and draped in appropriate manner for surgery in the oropharyngeal area. A McIvor mouth gag was placed to allow for visualization of the tonsils. Attention was first focused on the left tonsil. Under loupe magnification, the left tonsil was removed in its entirety from a superior to an inferior direction with needlepoint Bovie. Hemostasis was achieved in spots with suction cautery. A similar procedure was then performed on the right tonsil. Attention was then focused on the uvula and soft palate. After determining the appropriate amount of tissue to be removed, the area was infiltrated with 1% Xylocaine with 1:100,000 units of epinephrine. Then the mucosa and submucosal tissue of the soft palate and uvula were removed utilizing the needlepoint Bovie. The uvula was then split in the midline to create two uvula-palatal flaps. These flaps were then sutured in a superior and lateral direction with interrupted 3–0 chromic sutures in a figure-of-eight as well as simple closure. The area was then irrigated with saline. Subsequent reinspection showed no active bleeding. The tension on the mouth gag was then released. Reinspection showed no active bleeding. The mouth gag was then removed. The patient tolerated the procedure well, there was no break in technique, and the patient was extubated and taken to the postanesthesia care unit in good condition.

FLUIDS ADMINISTERED: 1600 ml of RL.

ESTIMATED BLOOD LOSS: Less than 50 ml.

PREOPERATIVE MEDICATION: 1 gram Ancef and 12 mg Decadron IV.

Pathology Report Later Indicated: Hypertropic tissue of uvula and tonsil.

CPT Code(s): _42145 , 42826_

ICD-9-CM Code(s): _327.23 , 474.00 , 528.9_

ICD-10-CM Code(s): _____

Abstracting Questions

1. Is the tonsillectomy reported in this case? _yes_

2. What other structure is considered when coding a tonsillectomy? _none adenoids_

3. What other factor affects the tonsillectomy code? _Age_

4. How many codes are required to report the remaining work? _1_

5. Recurrent tonsillitis would also be considered what? _chronic_

Case 44: Uvulopalatopharyngoplasty

OPERATIVE REPORT

LOCATION: Outpatient, Hospital

PATIENT: Lori Green

PREOPERATIVE DIAGNOSIS: Severe obstructive sleep apnea.

POSTOPERATIVE DIAGNOSIS: Same.

SURGEON: Jeff King, MD

PROCEDURE PERFORMED: Uvulopalatopharyngoplasty (UPPP).

OPERATIVE NOTE: This is a 31-year-old patient who was seen in the office and diagnosed with the above condition. Decision was made after consultation with the patient after explanation of the risks and benefits to undergo the above-named procedure.

She was admitted through the Same Day Surgery Program and taken to the operating room, where she was administered a general anesthetic by intravenous injection and was then intubated endotracheally. The Jennings gag was placed in the mouth and expanded. This was secured to the Mayo stand. The palate was examined. The proposed amount of tissue to trim was identified. We then used electrocautery and trimmed off the distal palate and uvula. We then cut trenches on either lateral side with the same electrocautery. The free margins of the palate were then reapproximated using interrupted 3–0 Vicryl suture. We then injected the area with 0.5% Marcaine with epinephrine; approximately 2 cc was used. The patient was then allowed to recover from general anesthetic and was taken to the postanesthesia care unit in stable condition. There were no complications during this procedure.

Pathology Report Later Indicated: Benign tissue.

CPT Code(s): _____42145_____

ICD-9-CM Code(s): _____327.23_____

ICD-10-CM Code(s): _____

Case 45: Myringotomy and Tympanostomy

OPERATIVE REPORT

LOCATION: Outpatient, Hospital

PATIENT: Casey Pullman

PREOPERATIVE DIAGNOSES
1. Chronic otitis media with effusion.
2. Bilateral eustachian tube dysfunction.
3. Conductive hearing loss.

POSTOPERATIVE DIAGNOSES: Same.

SURGEON: Jeff King, MD

PROCEDURE PERFORMED: Bilateral myringotomy and tympanostomy tube placement.

ANESTHESIA: General anesthetic by inhalational mask technique.

PROCEDURE IN DETAIL: Following informed consent from the patient's parent, the child was taken to the operating room and placed supine on the operating room table. The appropriate monitoring devices were placed on the patient. General anesthesia was induced. It was maintained by inhalational mask technique. The right ear was initially evaluated with the operating microscope. Wax was removed. A radial incision was made at the 6-o'clock position on the right tympanic membrane. A large amount of thick mucoid effusion was suctioned. A tube was placed. Topical antibiotic drops were then applied.

The left ear was then evaluated. Wax was removed. A radial incision was made at the 6-o'clock position on the left tympanic membrane. A large amount of thick mucoid effusion was suctioned from behind the left tympanic membrane. A tube was placed. Topical antibiotic drops were then applied.

The patient was then allowed to recover from general anesthesia. He will go home with a prescription for Ciprodex, 4 drops to each ear twice a day for 3 days. He will follow up in 2 to 3 weeks.

Pathology Report Later Indicated: Benign serous fluid.

CPT Code(s): ~~69421-50~~, 69436-50

ICD-9-CM Code(s): 381.3, 381.81, 389.~~22~~ 06

ICD-10-CM Code(s): _____

Case 46: Septoplasty

OPERATIVE REPORT

LOCATION: Outpatient, Hospital

PATIENT: Morris Schultz

PREOPERATIVE DIAGNOSIS: Septal deviation.

POSTOPERATIVE DIAGNOSIS: Same.

SURGEON: Jeff King, MD

PROCEDURE PERFORMED: Septoplasty with submucosal resection.

OPERATIVE NOTE: This is a 27-year-old gentleman who was seen in the office and diagnosed with the above condition. The decision was made in consultation with the patient, after explanation of the risks and benefits to undergo the above-named procedure.

He was admitted through Same Day Surgery Department and taken to the operating room and was administered general anesthetic by intravenous injection and was intubated endotracheally. His nose was decongested with 4 cc of 4% cocaine solution on nasal pledgets. A small amount of Afrin was also used. The patient was draped in the usual fashion. The packing was then removed and the left septum was injected with 1% lidocaine with epinephrine. A left hemitransfixion incision was created with a Beaver blade and a mucoperichondrial flap was elevated on this side; this was extended posteriorly over the perpendicular plate of ethmoid and vomer, extended inferiorly over a septal spur. We then separated the bony and cartilaginous septum to elevate it on the opposite side. We elevated on either side of the maxillary crest. A 4-mm osteotome was used to remove this. A portion of inferior cartilage was also removed. Once this was completed we laid the mucosa back into position and the septum was nicely reduced. We closed the caudal hemitransfixion incision with interrupted 3–0 chromic suture. The septum was closed with 4–0 plain gut suture. Doyle splints were then placed on either side of the nose. The patient was then allowed to recover from the anesthesia and was taken to the postanesthesia care unit in stable condition. There were no complications during this procedure.

Pathology Report Later Indicated: Benign septal fragments and tissue.

CPT Code(s): __30520__

ICD-9-CM Code(s): __470__

ICD-10-CM Code(s): _____

Abstracting Questions

1. Is the submucosal resection separately reported? __no__
2. Is the deviated septum acquired or congenital? __acquired__

Case 47: Tonsillectomy and Adenoidectomy

OPERATIVE REPORT

LOCATION: Outpatient, Hospital

PATIENT: Glory Pleasant

PREOPERATIVE DIAGNOSIS: Chronic adenotonsillitis.

POSTOPERATIVE DIAGNOSIS: Chronic adenotonsillitis.

SURGEON: Jeff King, MD

PROCEDURE PERFORMED: Tonsillectomy and adenoidectomy.

OPERATIVE NOTE: Glory is a 22-year-old who was seen in the office and diagnosed with the above condition. The decision was made in consultation with the patient after explanation of the risks and benefits to undergo the above-named procedure.

The patient was admitted through the Same Day Surgery Program and taken to the operating room where she was administered a general anesthetic via intravenous injection. She was then intubated endotracheally. A Jennings gag was placed in the mouth and expanded. This was secured to the Mayo stand. Two red rubber catheters were placed through the nose and brought out through the mouth. These were secured with snaps. This was done to elevate the palate. A laryngeal mirror was placed in the nasopharynx. The adenoid tissue was visualized. The adenoid tissue was removed in a systematic fashion using suction cautery. Once this was completed, the red rubbers were released and brought out through the nose. The right tonsil was then grasped with Allis forceps and retracted medially. The capsule was identified laterally using electrocautery. The tonsil was removed from its fossa in an inferior to superior fashion. Once this was completed, the bed was inspected and no bleeding was noted. The left tonsil was then grasped with Allis forceps and retracted medially. Again, electrocautery was used to identify the capsule laterally. The tonsil was removed from its fossa in an inferior to superior fashion. Once this was completed, the bed was inspected and no bleeding was noted. Three tonsillar sponges soaked in 0.5% Marcaine with epinephrine were then placed in the nasopharynx and one in each tonsil bed. These were left in position for 5 minutes. At the end, they were serially removed. The beds were inspected and no further bleeding was noted. The gag was then released and removed from the mouth. The TM joint was checked. The patient was then allowed to recover from the anesthetic and taken to the postanesthesia care unit in stable condition. There were no complications during this procedure.

Pathology Report Later Indicated: Benign tissue.

CPT Code(s): _____42820_____

ICD-9-CM Code(s): _____474.02_____

ICD-10-CM Code(s): _____

Case 48: Tonsillectomy

OPERATIVE REPORT

LOCATION: Outpatient, Hospital

PATIENT: Vernon Piker

PREOPERATIVE DIAGNOSES: Chronic tonsillitis, tonsillar and adenoid hypertrophy.

POSTOPERATIVE DIAGNOSES: Same.

SURGEON: Jeff King, MD

PROCEDURE PERFORMED: Tonsillectomy and adenoidectomy.

ANESTHESIA: General endotracheal.

PROCEDURE IN DETAIL: Following informed consent from the patient's mother, this 4-year-old child was taken to the operating room and placed supine on the operating room table. The appropriate monitoring devices were placed on the patient, and general anesthesia was induced. He was orally intubated without difficulty. He was draped in the usual fashion. A mouth gag was carefully placed into the oral cavity and opened. A catheter was placed through the right nostril and brought out through the mouth and snapped so as to retract the soft palate. The nasopharynx was evaluated with a mirror. There was a small amount of hypertrophic adenoid tissue present, and under direct vision with the mirror, several sweeps of the adenoid curette were necessary to remove the majority of the adenoid tissue. Sponges were then placed into the nasopharynx to allow for hemostasis (control of blood). The left tonsil was then grasped with a straight Allis. With the cautery set at 12 watts on the coagulation mode, it was dissected out from superior to inferior by creating a plane between the tonsil and its muscular bed. It came out in one piece without any bleeding.

The right tonsil was then removed in an identical fashion to the left tonsil. There was no bleeding. The right and left tonsillar fasciae were then each injected with approximately 2 ml of Marcaine with epinephrine. The sponges were then removed from the nasopharynx. There was still a small amount of bleeding going on, and hence it was necessary to use the suction electrocautery to cauterize several points in the nasopharynx to allow for hemostasis (control of blood), which was achieved. Following this, there was no further bleeding. The catheter was then removed from the nose and the mouth gag removed from the mouth. Estimated blood loss was less than 5 ml. The patient was then allowed to recover from the general anesthetic. He was transferred to the recovery room in good condition. He tolerated the procedure well.

Pathology Report Later Indicated: Hypertrophic tissue.

CPT Code(s): _____42820_____

ICD-9-CM Code(s): _____474.02_____

ICD-10-CM Code(s): _____

Case 49: Myringotomy

OPERATIVE REPORT

LOCATION: Outpatient, Hospital

PATIENT: Dough Rami

POSTOPERATIVE DIAGNOSIS: Chronic and acute otitis media with persistent serous otitis.

POSTOPERATIVE DIAGNOSIS: Same.

SURGEON: Jeff King, MD

PROCEDURE PERFORMED: Bilateral myringotomy with tube placement.

OPERATIVE NOTE: The patient was seen in the office and diagnosed with the above condition. The decision was made in consultation with the patient and/or family to undergo the above-named procedure. The risks and benefits of surgery were discussed prior to the procedure, and informed consent was obtained.

The patient was admitted through the Same Day Surgery Department and taken to the operating room. The patient was administered a general anesthetic by inhalation. A speculum was inserted into the right ear; any obstructing wax was removed. The tympanic membrane was visualized.

An anterior-inferior incision was created. A PE tube was placed through the incision. Two drops of Cortisporin were applied. The speculum was removed and inserted in the opposite ear. Again, any obstructing wax was removed. The anterior-inferior portion of the drum was visualized. An incision was made in this position. A PE tube was placed through the incision and two drops of Cortisporin were applied. The speculum was removed. The patient was allowed to recover from the general anesthetic and was taken to the postanesthesia care unit in stable condition. There were no complications during this procedure.

MIDDLE EAR FINDINGS: Copious fluid bilaterally.

Pathology Report Later Indicated: Benign serous fluid.

CPT Code(s): _____ 69421-50   69436-50 _____

ICD-9-CM Code(s): _____ 381.10   381.01 _____

ICD-10-CM Code(s): _____

Case 50: Septoplasty and Turbinoplasty

OPERATIVE REPORT

LOCATION: Outpatient, Hospital

PATIENT: Cindy Todd

PREOPERATIVE DIAGNOSES
1. Deformity and obstruction of the nasal septum.
2. Hypertrophic inferior turbinates.

POSTOPERATIVE DIAGNOSES: Same.

SURGEON: Jeff King, MD

PROCEDURE PERFORMED: Septoplasty and inferior turbinoplasties.

FINDINGS: The patient had a severe nasal septal deformity into the left nasal passage with essentially complete occlusion of this side. The right inferior turbinate had become very hypertrophic, filling up the disparity.

PROCEDURE: After patient was placed under general anesthetic, the nose was cocainized and the septum was injected with 1% Xylocaine with epinephrine.

The face was prepped and draped in a sterile fashion. A left hemitransfixional incision was made, and the mucoperichondrium and periosteum were elevated off on the left-hand side. The incision was then made through the cartilage approximately 2 cm cephalad to the distal end, and then the mucoperichondrium and periosteum were elevated off on the right-hand side. The bent cartilage and perpendicular plate of the septum were removed. In the floor of the nose on the left-hand side, the patient had a very extensive bony spur and it had displaced the cartilage entirely off into the left-hand side. This bony spur was removed with a 4-mm chisel.

Once removed the septum floated freely and was able to be moved back into the midline. This still left a small amount of curvature now into the right nasal passage, but I believe at this point it should not cause significant obstruction. The right nasal passage was suctioned and cleaned well. The left nasal passage was then open and straight. The septum was reattached anteriorly with a 4–0 nylon suture to hold it into position until it can glue down in the normal septal groove. The hemitransfixional incision was closed with interrupted 4–0 chromic suture. A Whipstitch was placed in the septum to bring the mucous membranes back together with 5–0 fast-absorbing suture. The inferior turbinates were then both injected full of 1% Xylocaine with epinephrine; following this, the Somnos machine was used, and 500 joules of energy were delivered to the superior part of both inferior turbinates and to the inferior part of both inferior turbinates to damage them and cause permanent retraction of the inferior turbinates. The nasopharynx was then suctioned and cleaned. Neo-Synephrine was placed in both sides of the nose. Telfa packing was placed; one pack in each side that was covered by bacitracin. The oral cavity was suctioned and cleaned well.

The patient was awakened from the anesthetic and returned to the recovery room in stable condition. Prognosis immediate and remote is good.

Estimated blood loss was 20 cc.

Pathology Report Later Indicated: Benign bony spur tissue.

CPT Code(s): _____

ICD-9-CM Code(s): _____

ICD-10-CM Code(s): _____

Abstracting Questions

1. How were the turbinates treated? _____

2. Does the method affect code selection? _____

Case 51: Bronchoscopy

OPERATIVE REPORT

LOCATION: Outpatient, Hospital

PATIENT: Anthony Radel

PREOPERATIVE DIAGNOSIS: Bilateral lower lobe ground-glass opacities and infiltrates consistent with possible interstitial lung disease.

POSTOPERATIVE DIAGNOSIS: Same.

SURGEON: Gregory Dawson, MD

PROCEDURE PERFORMED: Bronchoscopy.

Informed consent was obtained prior to the procedure. The patient was explained the risks, benefits, complications, and other options of the procedure.

Prior to the procedure, the patient was given codeine along with atropine to decrease the heart rate and suppress the cough reflex.

PROCEDURE: Topical anesthesia was applied with local lidocaine spray and also intranasal cocaine mix for the local vasocongestion and for local anesthesia. The procedure was performed in the fluoroscopy unit. The bronchoscope was introduced through the nostril and negotiated into the upper airway. The vocal cords were visualized. Vocal cords were moving equally with phonation and respiration. There was no abnormality found in the upper airway. Then the bronchoscope was negotiated through the vocal cords into the trachea and along the major airways. The airways all seemed to be pretty normal actually. There was no inflammation there. There were no endobronchial lesions. All the major bronchi to tertiary branches were visualized, and no endobronchial lesions were noted. Right upper, middle, and lower lobe bronchi and right main to the subsegmental branches were visualized, and no endobronchial lesions were noted. Again, the left main, left upper lingula, and lower lobe branches of the subsegmental branches were visualized, and no endobronchial lesions noted. Airway mucosa was completely normal. The bronchoscope was wedged into the right lower lobe; specimens were collected with brushings, washings, and bronchioalveolar lavage; and transbronchial biopsies were performed from the right lower lobe and the right middle lobe in one side.

The patient tolerated it pretty well; actually, it was an uneventful procedure. He will be monitored in the recovery room for a couple of hours and then will be discharged.

During the procedure, blood pressure, oxygen saturation, and EKG were continuously monitored and were uneventful. There was minor oozing in the first lobe, but was able to be controlled with local epinephrine instillation. It was an uneventful procedure.

Pathology Report Later Indicated: Benign specimens from the right lower lobe.

CPT Code(s): _____

ICD-9-CM Code(s): _____

ICD-10-CM Code(s): _____

Abstracting Questions

1. What was done during the bronchoscopy? _____

2. Do the other procedures affect code selection? _____

3. What approach was used for the biopsies? _____

4. Does the actual lobe biopsied affect code selection? _____

Case 52: Nocturnal Polysomnogram Study

LOCATION: Outpatient, Hospital

PATIENT: Bernice Nolan

ENTRANCE DIAGNOSIS: Fatigue, microscopic angiitis, and hypoxia.

PHYSICIAN: Jeff King, MD

The patient began the study on room air at 2217 and her O_2 saturation was 930. She spent the entire night without any observable snoring, without any observable apnea, but this is intermittently observed, and she had no oxygen saturation below 920 when she was not walking. She did get to the bathroom once and when she came back it was 890 and 900, but that didn't really count for sleeping.

This patient does not have significant desaturation with sleep and therefore does not need oxygen therapy during the sleeping hours.

CPT Code(s): _____

ICD-9-CM Code(s): _____

ICD-10-CM Code(s): _____

Abstracting Questions

1. What section of CPT is referenced to report these services? _____

2. Does the documentation meet the criteria according to CPT for polysomnography? _____

3. The study was essentially normal; what diagnosis codes would be reported? _____

Case 53: Walking O₂ Desaturation Study

LOCATION: Outpatient, Hospital

PATIENT: Jeanine Lee

ENTRANCE DIAGNOSIS: Dyspnea.

PHYSICIAN: Jeff King, MD

The patient's O_2 saturation on room air was 94%. She was able to walk for 6 minutes without stopping and went 300 feet. The patient did drop her O_2 saturation to 85% and was titrated up to 3 liters a minute by nasal prongs to keep the O_2 saturation above 88%. Borg scale was 0 throughout. The fastest heart rate recorded was 101.

The patient has reasonable exercise tolerance and does require oxygen at 3 liters a minute while walking.

CPT Code(s): _____

ICD-9-CM Code(s): _____

ICD-10-CM Code(s): _____

Abstracting Questions

1. What type of medical specialty testing is this? _____

Case 54: Pulmonary Function Study

LOCATION: Outpatient, Hospital

PATIENT: Brad Nord

PHYSICIAN: Gregory Dawson, MD

ENTRANCE DIAGNOSIS: Hypoxia, short of breath walking more than 100 yards, wheezes, 58.5 pack-year history of smoking, gave good effort; however, because he has a hip fracture, we could not get him in the body box, so we could not get most of the test.

INTERPRETATION
1. Flow volume loop shows significant concavity toward the volume axis, well-preserved inspiratory limb, and reduced flow rates of a significant degree.
2. There is no statistical significant change after bronchodilator.
3. Plethysmographic lung volumes could not be done.
4. Single-breath lung volumes are normal.
5. There is evidence of dynamic airway collapse (air trapping), which can be seen with obstructive disease.
6. DLCO was only 24% of predicted, which is quite reduced, suggesting reduced alveolar capillary membrane surface area and/or V/Q mismatching.
7. Prebronchodilator flow rates show a pattern consistent with obstructive disease of a moderate degree.
8. Post bronchodilator values show no significant change and the same conclusions can be reached.
9. The MVV is actually normal pre and post bronchodilator and between that and only a mildly abnormal FEV_1. I would expect only a mildly abnormal exercise tolerance.
10. Airway resistance could not be done.

The DLCO is reduced way out of proportion to reduction in flow rates, as is the patient's complaint of being short of breath walking less than 100 yards. It does not match the patient's defects seen on spirometry. Other causes should be looked for. Clinical correlation should, of course, be used.

CPT Code(s): _____

ICD-9-CM Code(s): _____

ICD-10-CM Code(s): _____

Abstracting Questions

1. Can this study be reported with only one code? _____

2. Does the pre- and post-bronchodilator administration affect spirometry code selection? _____

3. What do the following represent? _____

   a. DLCO _____

   b. MVV _____

   c. FEV _____

4. Is the measurement of the carbon monoxide reported separately from the spirometry? _____

5. Was there evidence of air trapping, determined via thoracic gas volume testing? _____

6. How do the "could not be done" procedures affect coding? _____

7. Is a definitive diagnosis determined? _____

Case 55: Right Chest Tube Placement

LOCATION: Outpatient, Hospital

PATIENT: Peter Nelson

EXAMINATION OF: Ultrasound-guided placement of a right chest tube.

PHYSICIAN: Gregory Dawson, MD

CLINICAL SYMPTOMS: Right pleural effusion.

ULTRASOUND-GUIDED PLACEMENT OF RIGHT CHEST TUBE: Informed consent was obtained. The patient was sat upright and his right back was prepped and draped in the usual sterile fashion. Skin and subcutaneous tissues were infiltrated with 1% lidocaine. Under ultrasound guidance, a 5 French Yueh catheter was placed into the right pleural fluid. Sixty milliliters of fluid was aspirated and sent to the lab for requested analysis. Over a 0.035 Amplatz guidewire, the Yueh catheter was exchanged for an 8.5 French Dawson-Mueller pigtail catheter. The catheter was secured to the skin with 2–0 Ethilon suture. The drainage catheter was placed to Pleur-evac suction.

The patient received conscious sedation. Signs were monitored throughout the exam. He tolerated the procedure well and left in stable condition.

Pathology Report Later Indicated: Normal right pleural fluid.

CPT Code(s): _____

ICD-9-CM Code(s): _____

ICD-10-CM Code(s): _____

Abstracting Questions

1. Could this procedure be considered a Thoracostomy? _____

2. Does the utilization of water seal affect the code reported? _____

3. Is the ultrasound guidance separately reported? _____

Case 56: Bronchoscopy

OPERATIVE REPORT

LOCATION: Outpatient, Hospital

PATIENT: Rick Sims

SURGEON: Gregory Dawson, MD

PROCEDURE PERFORMED: Bronchoscopy.

INDICATIONS: Right-sided lung collapse. Rule out endobronchial obstruction or mucous plug.

Informed consent was obtained from the patient and the family members prior to the procedure. The patient is not intubated. He was given topical anesthesia with lidocaine to the nose, as well as cocaine mix. The patient did have significant coagulopathy with nasal oozing present on the right side of nostril. With lidocaine administration the patient was significantly numbed up, and then going through the nasal cavity the bronchoscope was introduced into the right nostril and negotiated into the upper airway. The vocal cords were visualized. The vocal cords were moving equally with phonation and respirations. The secretions in the back of the throat in the posterior pharyngeal region were suctioned out through the bronchoscope, and subsequently the bronchoscope was introduced through the vocal cords and into the trachea and left upper lobe, and lingula up to subsegmental branches were visualized. No endobronchial lesions were noted on the left side. On the right side I did not find any mucous plugging but some blood-tinged secretions coming from the upper airway through the nose. They were frequently suctioned out. There was extensive compression of the right middle and lower lobe bronchi present suggestive of extensive compression probably from pleural effusion outside. The samples were collected for the infectious etiology with bronchial washings. The patient tolerated the procedure pretty well. His oxygen had to be supplemented to high amount F_{IO_2} through the mask during the bronchoscopy procedure. The patient tolerated the procedure well.

Pathology Report Later Indicated: Uncertain findings.

CPT Code(s): _____

ICD-9-CM Code(s): _____

ICD-10-CM Code(s): _____

Abstracting Questions

1. How is the pathology report's "uncertain findings" reported? _____

Case 57: Swan-Ganz Insertion

OPERATIVE REPORT

LOCATION: Outpatient, Hospital

PATIENT: Scott Nay

SURGEON: Ronald Green, MD

PROCEDURE PERFORMED: Placement of a pulmonary arterial (Swan-Ganz) catheter.

INDICATION: Monitoring of the patient's severe hypotension.

PROCEDURE: After the procedure and the potential complications were explained and consent was obtained from the patient's family, the patient was prepped for the placement of a pulmonary arterial catheter. The patient already had a pulmonary arterial catheter sheath in place.

The area had previously been sterilized with a Chloraprep and sterile drapes. The catheter was flushed and tested. The balloon tip was also found to be intact. The catheter was then inserted into the sheath until about the 20-cm mark, after which the balloon tip was inflated. The catheter was then slowly advanced into the superior vena cava into the right atrium through the tricuspid valve through the right ventricle, through the pulmonic valve, and into the pulmonary artery. Pulmonary artery occlusion was achieved at around 48 cm on the catheter. Central venous pressure, right atrial pressures, right ventricular pressures, pulmonary arterial pressures, as well as pulmonary arterial occlusions pressures were measured throughout. Insertion of the catheter was guided by the transduced waveforms. Once the catheter was in place, the cover sheath was then pulled out and the catheter secured.

The patient tolerated the procedure well. There were no acute complications. A chest x-ray had been requested to confirm correct placement of the catheter.

CPT Code(s): _____

ICD-9-CM Code(s): _____

ICD-10-CM Code(s): _____

Abstracting Questions

1. What was the ultimate destination for the insertion of this catheter? _____

2. Was this a diagnostic or therapeutic catheterization? _____

Chapter 8
General Surgery

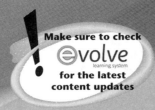

Make sure to check evolve *learning system* **for the latest content updates**

Case 58: Circumcision

OPERATIVE REPORT

LOCATION: Outpatient, Hospital

PATIENT: Allen Nam

PREOPERATIVE DIAGNOSIS: Phimosis.

POSTOPERATIVE DIAGNOSIS: Circumcision.

SURGEON: Paula Smithson, MD

PROCEDURE PERFORMED: Circumcision.

This 10-day-old young fellow was placed on a standard circumcision board. He was prepped in the standard procedure with Betadine. We then used sucrose and a pacifier. A total of 0.5 cc of lidocaine was injected at the 2-o'clock and 10-o'clock positions. He tolerated the procedure well. He did not even cry during it. We then used a Gomco clamp and removed the foreskin. Vaseline gauze was applied. There were no complications.

Pathology Report Later Indicated: Normal foreskin.

CPT Code(s): _54150_

ICD-9-CM Code(s): _V50.2   605_

ICD-10-CM Code(s): _____

Abstracting Questions

1. Does the age of the patient affect code selection? _no_

2. Does the technique affect code selection? _yes_

3. Is there a regional block used? _yes_

Case 59: Cystoscopy

OPERATIVE REPORT

LOCATION: Outpatient, Hospital

PATIENT: Eunice Nehring

SURGEON: Ira Avila, MD

The patient's maximal flow was 63.5 and average flow 37.5. Voided volume is 686 with residual urine of 150 cc. The CMG, EMG, and IRP show a lot of artifactual activity, but she was leaking throughout the procedure. Her first desire to void was 37 cc. Normal desire to void was 96 cc. Maximal capacity, however, was 161 cc. However, the information does not easily match the flow study where she had a much larger capacity with residual urine. The leak was noted very early on in the study and leaking continued throughout the study. The baseline shows a lot of artifacts but nothing that I can truly call uninhibited contractions of the bladder.

The patient had a cystoscopy performed today. She was prepared and draped in a sterile fashion. Following this, an endoscope was introduced through the urethra into the bladder. There is actually fairly good coaptation of the urethra at the bladder neck. Ureteral orifices were normal in size, shape, and position and well-developed interureteric ridge. There was no evidence of stone or tumor in the bladder. No trabeculation was present. There appeared to be a very mild subacute cystitis, but this was likely due to the fact that the patient had just had her urodynamic studies performed. The bladder was filled several times and emptied several times and re-examined. Examination of the mucosa revealed no evidence of any intersitial cystitis. With the bladder fairly well filled, I had the patient cough and bear down and she does have a lot of loss of urine from that position. This is relieved to some extent by pressure lateral to the urethra at the level of the bladder neck.

IMPRESSION:
1. Urinary incontinence with a predominant element of urinary stress incontinence.
2. Probable intrinsic sphincteric deficiency.
3. Elevated residual urine.
4. Some inconsistencies in urodynamic testing.

RECOMMENDATION: I gave the patient a prescription for Cipro following the procedure but she did not want to get that filled since she has lots of antibiotics she tells me at home, and she does have Augmentin and I suspect that is okay for her to take. I would recommend that at the time that she has her cystocele and rectocele repair and hysterectomy consideration be given to also placing a sling at the bladder neck to see if this could overcome her urinary incontinence. I told her about the elevated residual urine and discussed with her timed voiding and double voiding to try and get that bladder to empty better. The patient, if she has her operative procedure, is at a bit of a risk for urinary retention postoperatively, and I talked to her about the fact that if she has those procedures done, she may require intermittent self-catheterization for a while until it all balances out.

CPT Code(s): _____52000_____

ICD-9-CM Code(s): ____625.6_____

ICD-10-CM Code(s): _____

Abstracting Questions

1. Is this a diagnostic or surgical procedure? _Diagnostic_____

2. Is there a specific incontinence code to be reported? _yes_____

Case 60: Hernia Repair

OPERATIVE REPORT

LOCATION: Outpatient, Hospital

PATIENT: Thad Mark

PREOPERATIVE DIAGNOSIS: Left inguinal hernia.

POSTOPERATIVE DIAGNOSIS: Left indirect inguinal hernia.

SURGEON: Loren White, MD

PROCEDURE PERFORMED: Left inguinal hernia repair with large Prolene hernia graft.

ANESTHESIA: General.

INDICATION: The patient is a 32-year-old gentleman with a symptomatic left groin hernia, who presents today for elective repair, understands surgery and the risk for bleeding, infection, possible damage to the spermatic cord, and possible postoperative fluid collections, and he wishes to proceed.

PROCEDURE: The patient was brought to the operating room, placed under general anesthesia, and prepped and draped sterilely with Betadine solution. A left groin incision was made with a #10 blade, and dissection was carried down through subcutaneous tissues using electrocautery. External oblique was identified and opened along its fibers down to the external ring. Spermatic cord was isolated and looped with a Penrose drain. Hernia sac and cord lipoma were dissected free from the cord. These were reduced. A large Prolene hernia system patch was then placed with the underlay patch going through the patulous internal ring and lying underneath the transversalis fascia. The overlay patch was then tacked superiorly to the conjoined tendon, inferiorly to the inguinal ligament and medially to the fascia overlying the pubic tubercle. We had cut a slit in the overlay patch so that the cord could exit through. The external oblique was then closed with a running 3–0 Vicryl. We anesthetized the wound with 30 cc of 0.5% Sensorcaine with epinephrine solution and closed the skin with subcuticular 4–0 undyed Vicryl. Steri-Strips and sterile Band-Aids were applied. All sponge and needle counts were correct. He tolerated this well and was taken to the recovery room in stable condition.

Pathology Report Later Indicated: Mesothelial-lined fibrovascular tissue with skeletal muscle, consistent with left inguinal hernia.

CPT Code(s): _____49505 – Lt_____

ICD-9-CM Code(s): _____550.90_____

ICD-10-CM Code(s): _____

Abstracting Questions

1. Is the repair done open or via a scope? _____open_____

2. Does the location of the hernia affect code selection? _____yes_____

3. Does age affect code selection? _____yes_____

4. What three other factors affect code selection? _____initial, recurring, reduced_____

5. Is the mesh repair reported separately? _____no_____

6. What factors affect the diagnosis coding? _____age, location_____

Case 61: Removal of Dialysis Catheter

OPERATIVE REPORT

LOCATION: Outpatient, Hospital

PATIENT: Jane Lange

PREOPERATIVE DIAGNOSIS: Infected peritoneal dialysis catheter.

POSTOPERATIVE DIAGNOSIS: Same.

SURGEON: Loren White, MD

PROCEDURE PERFORMED: Removal of infected peritoneal dialysis catheter.

INDICATION: This is a 61-year-old female who has a peritoneal dialysis catheter placement. The wound has become infected and the catheter itself infected. It needs to be removed. We have discussed her diagnosis as well as the recommended procedure and the risks involved. She understands and wishes to proceed.

DESCRIPTION OF PROCEDURE: The patient was brought to the operating theater and placed in the supine position on the operating table. After receiving some IV sedation, she was prepped and draped in a sterile fashion. The infraumbilical incision site was all infiltrated with 0.5% Marcaine with epinephrine as well as the tunnel tract of the catheter. We then opened up the incision the full length. This had been partially opened before. We completed the opening with a #15 blade. The catheter was identified and easily dissected out. It was clamped. It was transected. A clamp was left on the side that went into the abdominal cavity. We then extracted the catheter out. This came out with ease. This was the subcutaneous portion. We then opened up the fascia just a little bit right around the cuff. We dissected things around here and made sure the entire cuff was removed. This was then handed off the table as specimen. We then closed the fascia defect with two interrupted sutures of 2–0 Vicryl. Care was taken to be sure that we got full fascia but did not incorporate any intra-abdominal contents. These were secured. The wound was irrigated and necrotic debris was debrided. Hemostasis was present. It was packed open with moistened 4 × 4 gauze. This probably took about half of it. We put the corner of a dry 4 × 4 up into the tunnel tract at the skin exit site. Sterile dry 4 × 4s were placed over this. The patient tolerated the procedure well and went to the recovery room in stable condition.

I met with the patient's husband postoperatively and discussed the operative findings with him.

CPT Code(s): _____49422_____

ICD-9-CM Code(s): _____996.68_____

ICD-10-CM Code(s): _____

Abstracting Questions

1. What is the location of the catheter? ___peritoneal___
2. What category of diagnosis code is used? ___complication___
3. Does the infection affect diagnosis selection? ___yes___

Case 62: Catheter Removal

OPERATIVE REPORT

PATIENT: Sheryl Landgraff

LOCATION: Outpatient, Hospital

PREOPERATIVE DIAGNOSES
1. End-stage renal disease.
2. Nonfunctioning peritoneal dialysis catheter.

POSTOPERATIVE DIAGNOSES: Same.

SURGEON: Gary I. Sanchez, MD

PROCEDURES PERFORMED
1. Removal of old peritoneal dialysis catheter.
2. Insertion of new tunneled peritoneal dialysis catheter.

INDICATION: This is a 27-year-old female who has end-stage renal disease and is currently on hemodialysis. We had placed a peritoneal dialysis catheter for urgent peritoneal dialysis. This has functioned well for about the first 3 to 4 days and then all of a sudden stopped working. Radiology tried to reposition. This ended up in the right upper quadrant. It was then also noted that there was a "kink" in the peritoneal dialysis catheter. We tried to irrigate again the other day. We were unable to get this to work. We discussed her dialysis and discussed options. We discussed going to the operating theater and trying to open up the midline incision and try to reposition the catheter. If this did not work we would place a new catheter. The risks of the procedure including bleeding, infection, and injury to intestines and other intraabdominal structures were all discussed again with her. Expected postoperative course and recovery were also discussed. She understood and wished to proceed.

PROCEDURE: The patient was brought to the operating theater and placed in the supine position on the operating room table. After receiving a general anesthetic, she was prepped and draped in sterile fashion. We had prepped the peritoneal catheter itself, the external portion. There appeared to be a little bit of fluid draining from this. We then flushed 20 cc of heparinized saline. There seemed to be a little bit of return at first. We started to aspirate things here. Then it was noted that there was fibrinous debris within the catheter. We continued aspiration until we were able to retrieve this. We then handed this off the table as a specimen to go for cultures. It was thought perhaps this is what was actually causing the obstruction. We flushed things out again, but we would only get a little bit of return. We would put about 20 cc in and get about 5 cc back each time. Even when we put in 40 cc, we would only get 5 cc back. Therefore it was decided that we needed to still further investigate this. Of course, the catheter was also in the right side of the abdomen into the right lower quadrant. It was not down in the pelvis. Incision was made in the vertical midline below the umbilicus. This was at the old incision site. Dissection was carried down to the fascia. There was resolving hematoma here. This was all cleaned out. Soft tissues were debrided. As we opened up the fascia I could not really identify any specific kinking or twisting here. Once we got this opened up, though, we pulled the catheter up. I decided at this time since there was some of this debris within the catheter and I was not 100% sure that this was not an infection I did remove it. My suspicions for this being an infection were quite low, however. Otherwise I would not even have put another catheter in. There was no purulent fluid within the cavity. There was just this fibrinous plug in the catheter. We removed the other catheter by withdrawing it out externally through the subcutaneous tissues and out through the skin without really any difficulty. We then took a new Quentin peritoneal dialysis catheter. This was placed with ease into the pelvis. The patient had been placed in Trendelenburg position. The patient was then flattened out. We then closed the fascia with 0 Vicryls in interrupted fashion. One of the Vicryls that was adjacent to the peritoneal dialysis catheter was used to "snag" into the cuff to help secure this in place. We made sure that all the sutures were not incorporating bowel or other structures. The sutures were then secured. The wound was irrigated out with Bacitracin solution. We flushed the catheter before closing the fascia as well as again after closing the fascia. This flushed easily and drained out easily also. We then made a new counterincision site, but again in the left lower quadrant. This was just a little bit higher and a little bit more lateral. I did not want to go in the exact same tract again. A Kelly clamp was used to create a curvilinear/arc tunnel. The catheter was pulled through this. This was through a new tunnel. The wound was irrigated out once again with Bacitracin solution. We also flushed out the old tract with the Bacitracin solution. We then closed the subcutaneous tissues around the catheter using a 3–0 Vicryl. We once again irrigated out the catheter. This flushed easily as well as retrieved easily. We did insert 40 cc of fluid and got 40 cc of heparinized saline back. The skin was then closed with a 4–0 Vicryl in running subcuticular fashion.

The old exit site was left open. Sterile dressings were applied. The patient tolerated the procedure well and went to the recovery room in stable condition.

CPT Code(s): _____ 94922 _____

ICD-9-CM Code(s): _____ 585.6 , 996.56 _____

ICD-10-CM Code(s): _____

Abstracting Questions

1. Are the removal and insertion of the replacement catheter both reported? ___ no _____

2. Is the diagnosis coding for non-functioning catheter reported differently than an infected catheter?

   ___ yes _____

Case 63: Cholangiopancreatogram and Sphincterotomy

OPERATIVE REPORT

LOCATION: Outpatient, Hospital

PATIENT: Brenda Langford

PREOPERATIVE DIAGNOSIS: Severe abdominal pain and elevated liver enzymes.

POSTOPERATIVE DIAGNOSIS: Same.

SURGEON: Loren White, MD

PROCEDURES PERFORMED
1. Endoscopic retrograde cholangiopancreatogram.
2. Endoscopic retrograde pancreatic sphincterotomy with removal of sludge.

INDICATION: This is a 23-year-old white female who is admitted with severe abdominal pain and elevated liver enzymes. Her alkaline phosphatase was 120. Bilirubin 1.8. AST 42. ALT 282. Amylase normal at 18. Lipase normal at 1. The patient had an ultrasound that showed normal size ducts, but there was evidence for possible cholelithiasis. The patient's alkaline phosphatase has risen to 154 and bilirubin now to 4. AST down to 106. ALT down to 284. The patient continues to have pain.

PREOPERATIVE MEDICATION
1. Demerol 75 mg.
2. Versed 6 mg.
3. Atropine 0.4 mg IV.

FINDINGS: The Pentax video duodenoscope was inserted without difficulty into the oropharynx. The stomach was rapidly viewed, and no lesions were seen. The pylorus was intubated and the endoscope was advanced to the second duodenum. Immediately seen was a fairly normal-appearing ampulla. There was a slight amount of heme on the surface. The first duct cannulated was the pancreatic duct. The pancreatic head, body, and tail were normal in size and course. There were no filling defects. The next duct cannulated was the common bile duct. The common bile duct was normal in size. There were no filling defects initially seen, except perhaps one air bubble after sphincterotomy was performed. We did perform a pancreatic sphincterotomy because the patient had continued in pain and elevated/rising bilirubin. She was obese, and the fluoroscopic imaging was suboptimal because of this. The ducts were not dilated.

As mentioned, a 1-cm sphincterotomy was performed. We then inserted a 1-cm balloon and pulled the balloon through the opening four times and took occlusion cholangiograms each time. The first time we pulled the balloon through there was some sludge present, dark color material, but other subsequent films did not reveal any filling defects and no other sludge was pulled out. The patient tolerated the procedure well without sequelae.

IMPRESSION: Normal pancreatogram and normal cholangiogram without initially any stones. A 1-cm sphincterotomy was performed and sludge was removed.

PLAN: The patient will have her amylase and liver enzymes checked in the morning. She should be able to undergo an attempt at laparoscopic cholecystectomy in the morning.

CPT Code(s): _____43260_____

ICD-9-CM Code(s): _____769.00 794.8_____

ICD-10-CM Code(s): _____

Abstracting Questions

1. Is the sphincterotomy separately reported? ___YES_____

2. Is a definitive diagnosis determined? ___NO_____

Case 64: Cholecystectomy

OPERATIVE REPORT

LOCATION: Outpatient, Hospital

PATIENT: Josette Fox

PREOPERATIVE DIAGNOSIS: Acute cholecystitis with choledocholithiasis.

POSTOPERATIVE DIAGNOSIS: Acute cholecystitis with choledocholithiasis.

SURGEON: Loren White, MD

PROCEDURE PERFORMED: Laparoscopic cholecystectomy.

ANESTHESIA: General.

INDICATION: This is a 29-year-old-female who was admitted with acute cholecystitis and elevated liver function tests. These levels continued to climb, and she underwent ERCP. They retrieved stones, and she presented today for elective laparoscopic cholecystectomy. She understands the risks for bleeding, infection, damage to the biliary system, and conversion to open procedure and she wishes to proceed.

PROCEDURE: The patient was brought to the operating room and placed under general anesthesia. A Foley catheter and orogastric tubes were inserted. She was prepped and draped sterilely. A supraumbilical skin incision was made with a #11 blade and dissection was carried down through subcutaneous tissues bluntly. The midline fascia was grasped with a Kocher clamp and a 0 Vicryl suture was placed on either side of the midline fascia. A Veress needle was inserted in the abdominal cavity. Drop test confirmed placement within the peritoneal space. The abdomen was then insufflated with carbon dioxide. A 10-mm trocar port and laparoscope were introduced showing no damage to the underlying viscera. Under direct vision, 3 additional trocar ports were placed, 1 upper midline 10 mm and 2 right upper quadrant 5 mm. The gallbladder was grasped and elevated from its fossa, and the cystic duct and artery were dissected free, doubly clipped proximally and distally before dividing them with Hook scissors. The gallbladder was then shelled from its fossa using electrocautery. It was very inflamed and edematous. We then brought it up and out of the upper midline incision.

We irrigated the abdomen with saline until returns were clear. We took a good look at the liver bed, there was no evidence of bleeding and clips were in good position. We removed all trocar ports under direct vision with no evidence of bleeding and closed the supraumbilical port site fascial defect with a single interrupted 0 Vicryl suture. The skin at all port sites was closed with subcuticular 4–0 undyed Vicryl. Steri-Strips and sterile Band-Aids were applied.

All sponge and needle counts were correct. Prior to leaving the operating room, the wounds were anesthetized with a total of 30 cc of 0.5% Sensorcaine with epinephrine solution.

Pathology Report Later Indicated: Consistent with choledocholithiasis.

CPT Code(s): _47562_

ICD-9-CM Code(s): _574.30_

ICD-10-CM Code(s): _____

Abstracting Questions

1. What is the approach for this procedure? _laproscopic_

2. What factor determines fifth digit for diagnosis? _acute & not acute_

3. Does the location of the stone affect the diagnosis coding? _yes_

Case 65: Dissection and Excision of Lymph Node

OPERATIVE REPORT

LOCATION: Outpatient, Hospital

PATIENT: Joy Froese

PREOPERATIVE DIAGNOSIS: Right upper neck cervical lymphadenopathy.

POSTOPERATIVE DIAGNOSIS: Same.

SURGEON: Gary I. Sanchez, MD

PROCEDURE PERFORMED: Dissection and excision of right upper neck deep jugular lymph nodes.

ANESTHESIA: General endotracheal anesthesia.

INDICATION: A 22-year-old female with persistently enlarged right upper neck deep jugular lymph nodes. The patient is now here for surgical treatment.

DESCRIPTION OF PROCEDURE: After consent was obtained, the patient was taken to the operating room and placed on the operating room table in the supine position.

After an adequate level of general endotracheal anesthesia was obtained, the patient was turned and draped in an appropriate manner for surgery on the right upper neck area.

The patient's right neck was prepped with Betadine prep and then draped in a sterile manner. A curvilinear incision was marked in the upper neck area approximately two fingerbreadths below the mandible. The area was then infiltrated with 1% Xylocaine with 1:100,000 units epinephrine. Under loupe magnification, sharp dissection was carried down through skin and subcutaneous tissue. Superior and inferior subplatysmal flaps were then elevated. Dissection was then carried anterior to the sternocleidomastoid muscle. The carotid sheath was identified. The enlarged lymph nodes were noted to be adjacent to the internal jugular vein. As such, with meticulous dissection, this was dissected. There appeared to be several large lymph nodes that were dissected away and sent as specimen. The spinal accessory nerve was identified and preserved. Hemostasis was achieved with silk ties as well as bipolar cautery. The area was then irrigated with saline. Subsequent reinspection showed no active bleeding. The wound was then closed in layers over a quarter-inch Penrose drain. The platysma and subcutaneous tissues were approximated with interrupted 4–0 Vicryl suture. The skin was approximated with a subcuticular closure of 5–0 Prolene. Benzoin and Steri-Strips were applied. Dressing of fluffs and Kerlix was then placed. The patient tolerated the procedure well, and there was no break in technique. The patient was extubated and taken to the postanesthesia care unit in good condition.

FLUIDS: 1100 ml RL.

ESTIMATED BLOOD LOSS: Less than 50 ml.

PREOPERATIVE MEDICATION: 1 gram Ancef and 12 mg Decadron IV.

Pathology Report Later Indicated: Tissue consistent with lymphadenopathy.

CPT Code(s): _____ 38542 - Rt _____

ICD-9-CM Code(s): _____ 785.6 _____

ICD-10-CM Code(s): _____

Abstracting Questions

1. Does the location of the lymph nodes affect code selection? _____ yes _____

2. Was this a radical excision? _____ no _____

Case 66: Aspiration and Biopsy

OPERATIVE REPORT

LOCATION: Outpatient, Hospital

PATIENT: Oliver Ganz

INDICATION:
1. Hypoproliferative anemia.
2. Development of lymphoma.
3. Aplastic anemia.
4. Myelodysplastic syndrome versus effective medications.

SURGEON: Edward Riddle, MD

PROCEDURE PERFORMED: Bone marrow aspiration and biopsy.

The need to perform the procedure, benefits, risks, and associated side effects were explained to the patient. Questions and concerns were answered. Informed consent has been obtained.

PROCEDURE: The patient was placed on his right lateral side. The left posterior iliac crest area was prepped by sterilizing the skin with Betadine. Local anesthesia with lidocaine was given. In addition, he received Versed 5 mg and fentanyl 50 mcg. After local anesthesia with lidocaine, a Jamshidi needle was inserted and approximately 4 ml of bone marrow aspirate and about 1.5 cm core biopsy were obtained. The patient tolerated the procedure well without any significant side effects. The specimen will be evaluated for morphology, flow cytometry, and cytogenetics.

Pathology Report Later Indicated: Nonmalignant cells found in bone marrow.

CPT Code(s): _____ 38221 _____

ICD-9-CM Code(s): _____ 284.9   202.80 _____

ICD-10-CM Code(s): _____

Abstracting Questions

1. Are the aspiration and biopsy both reported? _____ yes _____

2. What conditions are reported for this biopsy? ____ needle _____

Chapter 9
Emergency Department

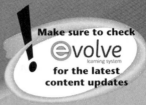

Make sure to check
evolve learning system
for the latest content updates

Report both the professional services for Dr. Sutton, a hospital employee, and facility services for the following cases.

Level 1—99281	Level 2—99282	Level 3—99283
1. Initial (triage) assessment 2. Suture removal 3. Wound recheck 4. Note for work or school 5. Simple discharge information	Interventions from previous level plus any of the following: 1. OTC med administration 2. Tetanus booster 3. Bedside diagnostic tests (stool hemoccult, glucometer) 4. Visual acuity 5. Orthostatic vital signs 6. Simple trauma not requiring x-ray 7. Simple discharge information	Interventions from previous level plus any of the following: 1. Heparin/saline lock 2. Crystalloid IV therapy 3. X-ray, one area 4. RX med administration 5. Fluorescein stain 6. Quick cath 7. Foley cath 8. Receipt of ambulance patient 9. Mental health emergencies (mild) not requiring parenteral medications or admission 10. Moderate complexity discharge instructions 11. Intermediate layered and complex laceration repair
Level 4—99284	**Level 5—99285**	**Critical care 99291, 99292**
Interventions from previous level plus any of the following: 1. X-ray, multiple areas 2. Special imaging studies (CT, MRI, ultrasound) 3. Cardiac monitoring 4. Multiple reassessments of patient 5. Parenteral[1] medications (including insulin) 6. Nebulizer treatment (1 or 2) 7. NG placement 8. Pelvic exam 9. Mental health emergencies (moderate). May require parenteral medications but not admission 10. Administration of IV medications [1]*not through the alimentary canal but rather by injection through some other route, such as subcutaneous, intramuscular, intraorbital, intracapsular, intraspinal, intrasternal, or intravenous*	Interventions from previous level plus any of the following: 1. Monitor/stabilize patient during in hospital transport and/or testing (CT, MRI, ultrasound) 2. Vasoactive medication 3. Administration (dopamine, dobutamine, multiple) nebulizer treatments (3 or more) 4. Conscious sedation 5. Lumbar puncture 6. Thoracentesis 7. Sexual assault exam 8. Admission to hospital 9. Mental health emergency (severe) psychotic and/or agitated/combative 10. Requires admission 11. Fracture/dislocation reduction 12. Suicide precautions 13. Gastric lavage 14. Complex discharge instructions	Interventions from any previous level plus any of the following: 1. Multiple parenteral medications 2. Continuous monitoring 3. Major trauma care 4. Chest tube insertion 5. CPR 6. Defibrillation/cardioversion 7. Delivery of baby 8. Control of major hemorrhage 9. Administration of blood or blood products

Case 67: Neck Pain

Assign an E code to indicate how the accident occurred.

LOCATION: Emergency Department

PATIENT: Betsey Anderson

PATIENT COMPLAINT: Neck pain.

PHYSICIAN: Paul Sutton, MD

HISTORY OF PRESENT ILLNESS: This is a 23-year-old woman who was involved in a motor vehicle accident today. She was a restrained front seat passenger in a car that had air bags that did deploy. She had a little bit of sharp neck pain after this accident. It has progressed a little bit more. It is actually in her upper shoulders. There is no numbness or tingling. She did not strike her head against anything and she has been doing well, but here at the emergency department she is placed in a C-collar and she is being evaluated in the presence of her mother.

PAST MEDICAL HISTORY: Her past medical history is negative.

PAST SURGICAL HISTORY: Her past surgical history is negative.

CURRENT MEDICATIONS: She is on no medications.

SOCIAL HISTORY: She does not smoke.

REVIEW OF SYSTEMS: Review of systems is as stated.

PHYSICAL EXAM: Temperature is 37.0, pulse rate is 109, respirations 61, blood pressure is 149/92. O_2 saturations are 99%. General appearance: Awake, alert, 23-year-old. HEENT: Head is normocephalic. C-collar is removed. I examined her posterior C-spine. There is no midline C-spine step-offs or crepitus or bony deformity. She is able to move her head through pain-free range of motion. She has some tightness in her upper shoulders. Only paraspinal tenderness is present. Neural exam: She is awake and alert. No dullness or tingling. She has excellent grip strength in her upper extremities.

EMERGENCY DEPARTMENT COURSE: The patient certainly will not need to have x-rays performed. She simply has a neck strain. I feel we can manage her as an outpatient with pain medications. She is provided Lorcet, Motrin, and also Norflex for pain control. She is agreeable with this plan.

ASSESSMENT: Acute neck strain, secondary to motor vehicle accident.

PLAN: The patient will be discharged. She is agreeable with the plan for follow-up. She understands my treatment regimen and again she understands that I do not believe she is a good candidate for an x-ray. I do not feel this will help her symptoms. She is aware that she may worsen tomorrow and she has appropriate instructions on how to deal with this.

CPT Code(s): _____

ICD-9-CM Code(s): _____

ICD-10-CM Code(s): _____

Abstracting Questions

1. Since this trauma case did not require x-rays, what level would it be? _____

2. What is the final finding for the patient's complaint? _____

3. How does the patient's position in the vehicle affect the E code? _____

Case 68: Back and Abdominal Pain

LOCATION: Emergency Department

PATIENT: Jodie Dvorak

PHYSICIAN: Paul Sutton, MD

SUBJECTIVE: This is a 32-year-old female in today for assessment of right low back pain and right-sided abdominal pain. The right flank pain started last night. It is hard to get comfortable. No prior similar symptoms. Standing up is actually a little better. No slips or falls. No trauma. No numbness or tingling. No nausea, vomiting, or diarrhea. Last normal menstrual period was several months ago. No abdominal pain was noted until my examination. No other significant symptomatology. She has no dysuria, hematuria, urgency, or frequency. No diarrhea, constipation, hematochezia. No upper GI symptoms. No respiratory tract symptoms.

PAST MEDICAL HISTORY: Reveals hyperprolactinemia. No other medical or surgical problems. No medications. No known drug allergies.

SOCIAL HISTORY: No tobacco utilization.

REVIEW OF SYSTEMS: Complete review of systems was undertaken and was negative.

OBJECTIVE: On examination today, temperature is 36, pulse 57, respirations 14; blood pressure 110/65, O_2 saturations 99% on room air. She is in no acute distress. Head and neck exam reveals normal TMs, canals, and ears. Nasal mucous membranes are slightly boggy. Oropharynx is unremarkable. Neck is supple. No cervical adenopathy. Chest is clear to auscultation and percussion with good air entry throughout. No rubs. No crackles. No wheezes. Heart sounds are normal. Rate and rhythm are normal. No rubs, clicks, or murmurs. No CVA tenderness. She is tender over the thoracolumbar junction on the right on palpation externally. It is reproducible, same place each time, about 1 inch to $1^1/_2$ inches lateral to the midline, just above the level of the thoracolumbar junction. Abdomen is tender throughout the right side. No guarding. No rebound. Good bowel sounds. No obvious organomegaly. Pelvic and rectal exam were deferred at this time. Skin is normal with no rash and no lesions. Hydration status is normal. KUB does not reveal any stones or lesions. It does reveal a lot of stool on the right-hand side. Urinalysis was completely negative. CBC reveals a white count of 8.5, normal differential cell count, and hemoglobin of 14. Normal indices. Platelet count of 350. HCG beta subunit was negative. Comprehensive metabolic panel to look at liver and gallbladder and electrolytes was all within normal limits, except for total protein being a little bit elevated.

IMPRESSION
1. Mechanical back pain. Treatment is steroid anti-inflammatories.
2. Abdominal pain secondary to constipation.

PLAN: Push fluids. Stool softeners. Follow up if signs or symptoms worsen or if any new problems are encountered or if symptom resolution is not forthcoming in a timely fashion.

CPT Code(s): _____

ICD-9-CM Code(s): _____

ICD-10-CM Code(s): _____

Abstracting Questions

1. What is the highest level of intervention provided for this patient? _____

2. Were more definitive diagnoses established from the presenting problems? _____

Case 69: Chest Pain

LOCATION: Emergency Department

PATIENT: Frances Miley

PHYSICIAN: Paul Sutton, MD

CHIEF COMPLAINT: Chest pain.

SUBJECTIVE: This is a 74-year-old female who presents to the emergency department complaining of chest pain. Apparently, this evening, she was talking to her son about his divorce. She then developed pain up her back, into her left arm and chest. She describes it as sharp and severe. Her Nitro did not help. One Nitro from our medics took the pain from a 10 to almost a 0. She has a history of chest pain and was placed on some p.r.n. Nitro. She was scheduled for a stress test, but she canceled it. She describes the pain as moderately severe, sharp in nature. It lasted approximately 1 hour.

PAST HISTORY: Significant for:
1. Degenerative joint disease.
2. Hypertension.

PAST SURGICAL HISTORY: Hip repair.

ALLERGIES: Sulfa.

FAMILY HISTORY: Negative for premature coronary artery disease.

SOCIAL HISTORY: She is a rare tobacco user and is not an alcohol user.

REVIEW OF SYSTEMS: Remarkable for the chest pain, as noted above, into the back and the arm, associated with diaphoresis and nausea. No vomiting. No fever, chills, or sweats.

CARDIOVASCULAR: As noted above.

RESPIRATORY, GI and GU: Negative.

OBJECTIVE: VITAL SIGNS: Stable. She generally appears well. She is nondiaphoretic. HEENT: Grossly benign and deferred. LUNGS: Mostly clear without rales, rhonchi, or wheezing. CARDIOVASCULAR EXAM: S1, S2 without obvious S3, murmur, or rub. CHEST WALL: Nontender. ABDOMEN: Soft. Bowel sounds are active. No masses, rebound, or rigidity.

LABORATORY: We did obtain an electrocardiogram, which is without hyperacute ST-T wave change. Blood work is remarkable for hemoglobin of 11.6. Basic metabolic panel is normal. CK and troponin are negative.

ASSESSMENT:
1. Chest pain.
2. Anemia.

PLAN: I have notified the patient's primary physician and he has graciously agreed to assume care and will be admitting the patient presently.

CPT Code(s): _____

ICD-9-CM Code(s): _____

ICD-10-CM Code(s): _____

Abstracting Questions

1. How does the admission to the hospital affect Professional Services? _____

2. How does the admission to the hospital affect Facility Services? _____

3. Was there a definitive diagnosis for the presenting problem of chest pain? _____

4. Are there any other diagnoses that should be reported? _____

Case 70: Foot Injury

Assign an E code to indicate how the accident occurred.

LOCATION: Emergency Department

PATIENT: Tanner Gray

PHYSICIAN: Paul Sutton, MD

SUBJECTIVE: This is a 4-year-old male who has history of reactive airway disease; he is on Singulair. He has no known allergies. He is up to date for immunizations. He presents to the emergency department with a history of injury to his left third and fourth toes when a bedroom TV dropped on his foot accidentally.

NEUROMUSCULOSKELETAL REVIEW OF SYSTEMS: He is not describing any paresthesias. Range of motion has been uncomfortable due to pain and the injury.

OBJECTIVE: He is afebrile, pulse 108, respiratory rate 30. Examination reveals a slight injury to the distal third toe with a possible slight fracture of the nail. This is minimal, however. The fourth toe has a partial nail avulsion. There is full range of motion, and the toes are neurovascularly intact.

X-ray of the left foot with emphasis on the distal third and fourth toe injuries is negative for gross bony abnormality.

ASSESSMENT: Left fourth and third toe injuries as described above with partial nail avulsion of the left fourth toe.

PLAN: These injuries were dressed with Bacitracin nonadherent dressing, 4 × 4s, and Kling wrap. We recommend ice, elevation, ibuprofen or Tylenol, and a follow-up for dressing change and wound check on Thursday or Friday with Dr. Lewis. His condition was stable at the time of discharge.

CPT Code(s): _____

ICD-9-CM Code(s): _____

ICD-10-CM Code(s): _____

Abstracting Questions

1. What is the highest level of intervention provided for this patient? _____

2. Are the different types of injuries reported for each toe? _____

3. Is more than one E code required? _____

Case 71: Leg Laceration

Assign an E code to indicate how the injury occurred.

LOCATION: Emergency Department

PATIENT: DeDe Clites

PHYSICIAN: Paul Sutton, MD

CHIEF COMPLAINT: Right leg laceration.

HISTORY OF PRESENT ILLNESS: A 59-year-old female presents with the chief complaint of a right leg laceration. The patient was at work today when a locker fell on top of her and she sustained blunt trauma to the right shin area. She cannot remember her last tetanus shot.

OBJECTIVE: She has a 4.0-cm flap laceration over the lateral aspect of the right mid shin. The full extent of this wound is seen. It is through the dermis into the subcutaneous fat but no underlying muscle involvement.

ASSESSMENT: Right leg laceration.

PLAN: This is cleansed with normal saline. One percent lidocaine with bicarb was used for local anesthesia. This was irrigated with saline and sutured first with 4–0 Vicryl a total of 1 suture in the dermis and then 5–0 Ethilon a total of about 10 mattress sutures in the skin. Suture removal in 10 days and a wound care sheet was given.

CPT Code(s): _____

ICD-9-CM Code(s): _____

ICD-10-CM Code(s): _____

Abstracting Questions

1. Would an E/M be reported? _____

2. What is the complexity of wound repair done? _____

3. Does body site affect code selection? _____

4. What is the other criterion for laceration repair code assignment? _____

Case 72: Left Lower Quadrant Pain

LOCATION: Emergency Department

PATIENT: Loretta Striker

PHYSICIAN: Paul Sutton, MD

SUBJECTIVE: The patient is a 65-year-old woman who presents to the emergency department. She initially saw my partner, and then care was turned over to me. We are just waiting for urinalysis results. Working diagnosis at this point was possible renal colic. The patient has stated the pain started this afternoon and worsened. She describes it mainly in the left lower quadrant. It radiates a little bit toward the left flank, sort of on the top of her left hip area on her side. She had two episodes of diarrhea today. She also carries a history of spastic colon for numerous years. She states that when that flares she usually has a little bit of low mid-back pain before she has a bowel movement. A lot of times it is mostly water, and then the pain goes away with that. This therefore does not feel like that. Her spastic colon has been flaring the last three weeks she tells me. She has had one ovary removed and she does not know which one. She has also had an appendectomy in the past. She has not noticed any discoloration to her urine. No dysuria, hematuria, or frequency.

EXAMINATION: Examination reveals pain to palpation in the left lower quadrant. No focal mass. No guarding. No CVA tenderness; we did review the KUB and it showed no obvious stones. However, there is a small radial opaque density across from L5, maybe 10 cm laterally. I think that is too far out to be the ureter. Some scattered stool and gas. Urinalysis showed 4 to 5 white cells, no red cells, and 2+ bacteria; this was on a sample with 1 to 2 epithelial cells. She had been given Tordal 60 mg IM. I checked on her and she states she still has pain, although it was better. I talked to her at length about possible diagnoses, including renal colic. I also talked about diverticulitis, which is difficult to say if she has that at this point. Also, possibly ovarian related such as a cyst, but I think that is not as likely either.

I talked to the patient about giving her some more pain medicine here and monitoring this, but she wanted to leave. I did request that she drink plenty of fluids, strain her urine, and follow up with her doctor this week. She said she was going to call him tomorrow. I told her that if her pain in any way changes or worsens tonight she should return. I sent her home with some Lorcet.

CPT Code(s): _____

ICD-9-CM Code(s): _____

ICD-10-CM Code(s): _____

Abstracting Questions

1. What is the highest level of intervention provided for this patient? _____
2. Were more definitive diagnoses confirmed after evaluation from presenting problems? _____

Case 73: Body Ache, Fever, and Headache

LOCATION: Emergency Department

PATIENT: Pearl Rumnick

PHYSICIAN: Paul Sutton, MD

CHIEF COMPLAINT: Body aches, fever, headache.

SUBJECTIVE: This 49-year-old female presents to the emergency department complaining of general body aches associated with headache, nausea, and cough, which has been occasional. She felt "yucky" last evening. She says she felt hot and cold. Again, slight cough associated with headache and chills. She describes the body aches as mild to moderate in severity. There are no other associated symptoms. No vomiting. She does admit to nausea and the cough.

PAST MEDICAL HISTORY: Hypertension, hyperlipidemia, depression, migraine, irritable bowel, avascular necrosis status post right and left hip surgery, ectopic pregnancy, appendectomy, tonsillectomy, adenoidectomy.

FAMILY HISTORY: Fairly unremarkable.

SOCIAL HISTORY: She is a widow, nonsmoker, and nondrinker.

REVIEW OF SYSTEMS: Remarkable for the hot and cold flashes, general myalgias, slight cough, headache, chills. No vomiting, some nausea.

PHYSICAL EXAMINATION: On physical exam, temperature is 38.4; vitals are otherwise stable. On exam, she is alert and oriented ×3. Neck is nontender with flexion. TMs and throat are benign. Neck is without adenopathy. Lungs are clear. Heart is without murmur. The abdomen is soft.

HOSPITAL COURSE: She was given Tylenol 1 gram p.o., an influenza swab was negative, and this was followed by some parenteral morphine and Vistaril, which afforded her some relief.

ASSESSMENT: Headache, fever.

PLAN: Reassurance, at this point. Conservative measures discussed. She is improved. Certainly to follow up in the emergency department for persistent or worsening symptoms; otherwise, on an as needed basis.

CPT Code(s): _____

ICD-9-CM Code(s): _____

ICD-10-CM Code(s): _____

Abstracting Questions

1. What is the highest level of intervention provided for this patient? _____

2. What diagnoses would be reported? _____

Case 74: Chest Congestion

LOCATION: Emergency Department

PATIENT: Dale Ray

PHYSICIAN: Paul Sutton, MD

This 33-year-old male presents to the emergency department for evaluation of chest congestion, cough, and chills.

HISTORY OF PRESENT ILLNESS: The patient is here in the emergency department describing symptoms, which started this past Sunday. He states he had a decreased appetite. He has had chills and shakes and he states that he has been feeling run down and tired. He has not had a fever, but states he does not always get a fever when he gets ill. He has been coughing and having quite a bit of chest congestion and he is increasingly worried about possibility of pneumonia. He had had some greenish phlegm drainage when he has coughed up recently and has had problems with pneumonia in the past. He did state that he had slight blood-tinged sputum once as well and for that reason he presents to the emergency department for evaluation. The patient's symptoms have been worsening since they began this past Sunday, and although he has been able to eat and drink he has had increasing fatigue. He just feels "foggy" and is worried that he may have something that would need treatment. He did note that he has received the flu shot.

PAST MEDICAL HISTORY: The patient's medical history includes previous urinary tract infections and pneumonia. He does have some muscle spasms.

MEDICATIONS: His medications include Baclofen, Singulair.

ALLERGIES: Bactrim.

SOCIAL HISTORY: The patient is a nonsmoker.

REVIEW OF SYSTEMS: His review of systems is negative for fevers. He has very mild headache. He denies any photophobia. No nausea or vomiting. He does not sense abdominal pain, leg pain, or dysuria or urinary symptoms and actually has a urostomy at this time as well. The patient has had some dyspnea and occasional palpitation, no dizziness. He states he has had swollen cervical lymph nodes. No skin rashes or lesions at this time. All other systems are reviewed and are negative.

EXAMINATION: General examination shows an awake, alert male who is oriented and cooperative. His vital signs in the emergency department show a temperature of 36.5, pulse 105, respiratory rate is 20, and blood pressure is 90/63. Saturations are 91% on room air. HEENT exam shows his head normocephalic and pupils reactive. Nares patent. Oropharynx is clear. He has midline trachea. Tracheostomy is in place. Neck is otherwise supple and nontender. Clavicles are nontender. He has coarse rhonchi in his lungs bilaterally, worse on the right than on the left. Slightly diminished air exchange is noted. His lungs are also remarkable for occasional wheeze. Heart is regular. Abdomen is soft at this time. Stoma appears pink and viable. He has urine output from the urostomy. His back does not have any evidence of breakdown or rash. His skin is warm and dry.

SUMMARY OF EMERGENCY DEPARTMENT COURSE: This 33-year-old male presents to the emergency department for cough with occasional sputum production and also had a little bit of blood-tinged sputum at one time as well. He does not have a fever and he is not appearing particularly short of breath at this time, but does have the history of pneumonia in the past. I inquired about previous antibiotic use and we noted that he has had a history of *Pseudomonas* pneumonia. He has just been treated about two weeks ago with a course of Cipro.

Here in the emergency department we did go ahead and obtain a urine culture, sputum cultures, CBC including a white count of 10.86, hemoglobin 13, platelet count 284 with 88.5% neutrophil, suggesting left shift. The metabolic panel is normal except for slightly low sodium at 135. His BUN is 20, creatinine of 0.8. Urinalysis showed 40 to 60 white cells, 20 to 30 red cells. Positive nitrites. Large leukocytes were also noted. This was obtained from the stoma and not the bag. We will send that for culture. We did review findings of chest x-ray, which showed right lower lung field radiopacity consistent with pneumonia. So we did get the blood gas, which showed a pH of 7.4. Pco_2 was 30. Po_2 was 57. So he does have some hypoxia with this. Because of his prior history of *Pseudomonas* pneumonia, we started him on ceftazidime 1 gram IV along with gentamicin 340 mg IV × 1. He was given albuterol nebulizer, which did seem to help him, and we continued him on oxygen here. Because of his comorbidities and his history of problems with significant pathogen and pneumonia here, we did admit the patient. The patient agrees to stay and is pleased to come into the hospital because of significant problems in the past.

ASSESSMENT: Acute right lower lobe pneumonia with hypoxia.

PLAN: We will certainly await the cultures for urinalysis. We did note the findings. He has already received his initial antibiotics here in the emergency department including ceftazidime and gentamicin. Blood cultures are pending at this point. He will be admitted to the floor for further evaluation and treatment. The patient is comfortable with that. His questions were answered. He is admitted in fair condition with the diagnosis of acute right lower lobe pneumonia with hypoxia.

CPT Code(s): _____

ICD-9-CM Code(s): _____

ICD-10-CM Code(s): _____

Abstracting Questions	

1. How does the admission to the hospital affect Professional Services? _____

2. How does the admission to the hospital affect Facility Services? _____

3. Were definitive diagnoses established after evaluation from presenting problems? _____

Case 75: Hematuria

LOCATION: Emergency Department

PATIENT: Neil Haugen

PHYSICIAN: Paul Sutton, MD

CHIEF COMPLAINT: Hematuria.

SUBJECTIVE: Pleasant 77-year-old male presents to the emergency room with hematuria. Notably, he was just recently discharged from the hospital with a similar type episode. He has had a recent TUNA procedure, which is basically a noninvasive procedure for BPH. He has a history of chronic renal insufficiency, glomeruli nephropathy, BPH, hyperlipidemia, hypothyroidism, hypertension, anemia, and retinopathy. He has had a bypass. He has noted gross blood started this morning. He does have a Foley catheter in place. He is on chronic hemodialysis and did have dialysis run this morning. There are no other associated symptoms or modifying factors. He says his pain is currently a 1. He denies any fever.

PAST MEDICAL HISTORY: As noted above.

FAMILY HISTORY: Noncontributory.

SOCIAL HISTORY: He is married; I believe a nonsmoker.

REVIEW OF SYSTEMS: No fever, positive for the hematuria. No chest pain. No increased shortness of breath.

PHYSICAL EXAMINATION: Vitals are stable. He appears markedly less than stated age. Lungs are clear. Heart is regular. The abdomen is soft. Extremities are unremarkable. Foley does show hematuria in the bag. We did obtain a CBC. Platelet count was slightly low at 76,000, hemoglobin 12, white count is normal. We did irrigate his three-way bag, which cleared the blood somewhat.

ASSESSMENT: Hematuria.

PLAN: The patient is certainly stable from a hemodynamic point of view and was discharged and is to follow up with his urologist.

CPT Code(s): _____

ICD-9-CM Code(s): _____

ICD-10-CM Code(s): _____

Abstracting Questions

---

1. What is the highest level of intervention provided for this patient? _____

Case 76: Fall

Assign an E code to indicate how the accident occurred.

LOCATION: Emergency Department

PATIENT: Floyd Gram

PHYSICIAN: Paul Sutton, MD

SUBJECTIVE: This is a 75-year-old male who comes to the ED with a history of falling last night, and he also fell about 10 days ago. The patient has been quite a bit weaker at home. He uses a walker for ambulation. He is having a much more difficult time lately according to his daughter and his wife. He has no pain in his bilateral rib area. He says he has had no hip pain and no lower extremity pain. Since the fall last night, he has got severe pain in the mid back area that is about an 8-9/10 severity and his wife feels he needs pain management. The patient has a history of kyphoplasties in the past due to compression fractures.

PAST MEDICAL HISTORY: Significant for chronic renal failure. He is on hemodialysis for that. He has also had a history of TURPs. He has a history of bypass surgery and a pacemaker. He has no history of hypertension, diabetes, or other problems. He has had gallbladder surgery and an appendectomy.

ALLERGIES: He has no known allergies.

SOCIAL HISTORY: He has a remote history of smoking, quit in 1961. He denies any alcohol use.

REVIEW OF SYSTEMS: Negative for fever, chills, sweats. He has had some weakness, but no fatigue. HEENT is negative for blurred or double vision. No hearing loss or ringing in the ears. Cardiovascular is negative for chest pain. Respiratory is negative cough, hemoptysis. He has had no dyspnea at rest or dyspnea on exertion. GI is negative for abdominal pain, nausea, or vomiting. GU is negative for dysuria or frequency of urination. There have been no muscle aches or pains. Skin is negative for rash. Neuro exam is intact, shows him in no depression. No memory problems, no thyroid problems, and no anemia or asthma.

OBJECTIVE: This is a 75-year-old male who appears to be in moderate to serious discomfort with back pain. Temperature is 36.5, pulse 114, respirations 24, blood pressure 128/78, oxygen saturations 99%. HEENT: Head is normocephalic, atraumatic. TMs are negative. PERRLA, EOMs are full. Oropharynx is unremarkable. Mucous membranes are moist. Neck is supple. There is no spinous process tenderness. Shoulders are nontender. Clavicles are nontender. Chest shows bilateral rales in both lung fields. There is tenderness in the left lateral chest wall area. The patient does have a dialysis catheter and tape in place in the right upper chest area. Cardiac: Normal S1 and S2 without murmur, rub, click, or gallop. Abdomen is soft, active bowel sounds, no guarding or rigidity. No tenderness to palpation of the abdomen.

Back shows some tenderness over the midthoracic spine to palpation. The lumbosacral spine and pelvis is nontender. Lower extremities show good pulses and no evidence of swelling. CBC was done and showed a white count of 3860 with hemoglobin of 12.5. Basic metabolic panel showed a BUN of 20 with a creatinine of 2.2. Thoracic spine and PA and lateral chest x-rays were done and showed no pneumothorax. The thoracic spine did show compression fractures at T3 and T8.

ASSESSMENT: New compression fractures at T3 and T8.

PLAN: We will see about doing a kyphoplasty today. This was done and this was not going to be feasible today due to the late time in the afternoon. He did recommend getting a bone scan and find out about the condition of his other vertebrae since he has had at least three previous kyphoplasties. The patient will be admitted for pain control and surgery.

CPT Code(s): _____

ICD-9-CM Code(s): _____

ICD-10-CM Code(s): _____

Abstracting Questions

1. How does the admission to the hospital affect Professional Services? _____

2. How does the admission to the hospital affect Facility Services? _____

3. Is there a more definitive diagnosis than back pain? _____

4. Are the vertebral fractures coded as traumatic or pathologic? _____

5. Is an E code assigned for the fall? _____

Chapter 10

Diagnostic Radiology

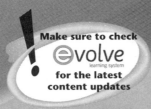
Make sure to check evolve learning system for the latest content updates

Case 77: Ultrasound, Carotid

LOCATION: Outpatient, Hospital

PATIENT: Kerry Redder

PHYSICIAN: Morton Monson, MD

Clinical history is history of left CEA. Follow-up showed stenosis on right. Patient had previous study.

Atherosclerotic plaque is identified on the right including hyperechoic and some hypoechoic plaque is seen. Atherosclerotic plaque is seen along the carotid bulb extending along the proximal internal carotid and proximal external carotid arteries. Peak systolic velocity right common carotid artery equals 74 cm/sec consistent with 50% to 75% stenosis. This is not significantly changed since previous value of 193 cm/sec. Peak systolic velocity right external carotid artery is somewhat elevated at 136 cm/sec. Previous value 89 cm/sec. IC/CC ratio 2.5. Right vertebral artery appears antegrade in flow.

Vessels on the left are noted to be somewhat tortuous. Obvious plaque is not identified on the left. Peak systolic velocity left common carotid artery equals 93 cm/sec, and left internal carotid artery equals 85 cm/sec. Peak systolic velocity left external carotid artery 101 cm/sec, and IC/CC ratio on the left 0.91. Left vertebral artery appears antegrade inflow.

IMPRESSION
1. Findings consistent with 50% to 75% stenosis right internal carotid artery. This has not significantly changed from prior study.
2. Somewhat elevated right external carotid artery is now seen with a peak systolic velocity of 136 cm/sec, suggesting some narrowing/stenosis there now.
3. Atherosclerotic plaque identified on the right as discussed above.
4. Vessels are tortuous on the left. No evidence of hemodynamically significant stenosis on the left. No obvious plaque identified.

CPT Code(s): _____

ICD-9-CM Code(s): _____

ICD-10-CM Code(s): _____

Abstracting Questions

1. When referencing the Index of the ICD-9-CM "stenosis," what else do you need to know? _____

2. What reference is made under "stenosis, artery, carotid" for further investigation? _____

3. How is the fifth digit assigned? _____

Case 78: Ultrasound, Pelvic and Transvaginal

LOCATION: Outpatient, Hospital

PATIENT: Peggy Brundle

PHYSICIAN: Morton Monson, MD

EXAMINATION OF: Pelvic and transvaginal sonogram.

HISTORY: Cramping.

FINDINGS: The uterus measures 5.3 × 5.0 × 3.8 cm. The endometrial stripe measures 0.7 cm in thickness. This patient is postmenopausal; therefore I assume this is an abnormal measurement unless the patient is on hormone replacement therapy. There are two ovoid anechoic foci within the lower uterine segment and cervix, which are likely due to nabothian cysts. The uterus itself does not demonstrate focal hypoechoic mass. Both ovaries are identified and are grossly normal. No adnexal masses. No adnexal free fluid. The right ovary measures 2.1 × 1.3 × 0.9 cm, and the left ovary measures 1.9 × 1.6 × 1.9 cm.

CPT Code(s): _____

ICD-9-CM Code(s): _____

ICD-10-CM Code(s): _____

Abstracting Questions

1. Are both the pelvic and transvaginal studies reported? _____
2. Is there a definitive diagnosis or is the presenting symptom reported? _____
3. Why would "nabothian cysts" not be reported? _____

Case 79: Ultrasound, Renal

LOCATION: Outpatient, Hospital

PATIENT: Sam Gage

PHYSICIAN: Morton Monson, MD

EXAMINATION OF: Renal sonogram.

CLINICAL SYMPTOMS: Chronic renal failure.

RENAL SONOGRAM: FINDINGS: Kidneys are relatively symmetric in size, shape, and appearance. The cortices do not appear atrophied.

The right kidney measures $10.2 \times 4.3 \times 5.5$ cm, and the left kidney measures $10.2 \times 4.3 \times 5.9$ cm. No evidence of masses or stones bilaterally. Prominent pyramids bilaterally. The bladder is moderately distended for this examination, and no postvoid images were obtained.

CPT Code(s): _____

ICD-9-CM Code(s): _____

ICD-10-CM Code(s): _____

Abstracting Questions

1. Is this a complete or limited exam? _____

Case 80: Ultrasound, OB

LOCATION: Outpatient, Hospital

PATIENT: Maria Zon

PHYSICIAN: Morton Monson, MD

EXAMINATION OF: Limited OB ultrasound.

CLINICAL SYMPTOMS: Preterm labor.

LIMITED OB ULTRASOUND: FINDINGS: A single active intrauterine gestation in longitudinal lie and cephalic presentation is identified. Average gestational age is 31 weeks 3 days. This represents interval growth of 23 weeks 1 day and chronologic growth of 22 weeks 3 days. Fetal heart rate is recorded at 128 beats per minute. Systolic/diastolic ratios of the umbilical artery on today's exam were measured at 4, 3.4, 3.4, which is within normal limits. Normal for 33 weeks would be 4.2 or less.

IMPRESSION: Normal interval growth and normal umbilical arterial ratio.

CPT Code(s): _____

ICD-9-CM Code(s): _____

ICD-10-CM Code(s): _____

Abstracting Questions

1. Does the gestational age affect code selection? _____

2. Was this a complete or limited exam? _____

3. Is this the initial or a follow-up exam? _____

4. Does the gestational age affect ICD-9-CM code selection? _____

5. What fifth digit is required for this case? _____

Case 81: Umbilical Arterial Doppler

LOCATION: Outpatient, Hospital

PATIENT: Crissy Snow

PHYSICIAN: Morton Monson, MD

EXAMINATION OF: Umbilical arterial Doppler.

CLINICAL SYMPTOMS: Hypertension complicating pregnancy.

UMBILICAL ARTERIAL DOPPLER: FINDINGS: Limited evaluation was performed. A single active intrauterine gestation is identified in longitudinal lie in cephalic presentation with fetal heart rate recorded at 121 beats/min. Relatively normal-appearing umbilical arterial waveform is present. Three umbilical artery Doppler tracings were done with systolic-to-diastolic ratio measured at 3, 2.9, 3.3. Normal systolic-to-diastolic ratio from 32 to 33 weeks would be less than 4.2. Previous umbilical arterial ratios were 3.2, 3.7, and 2.5 on 04/04/XX. The AFI on today's exam is measured at 9.6%, which places this between the 5th and 50th percentile.

CPT Code(s): _____

ICD-9-CM Code(s): _____

ICD-10-CM Code(s): _____

Abstracting Questions

1. How many code options are listed for this study? _____

2. What condition is complicating this pregnancy? _____

Case 82: Ultrasound, Fetal

LOCATION: Outpatient, Hospital

PATIENT: Shasta Hutton

PHYSICIAN: Morton Monson, MD

EXAMINATION OF: Biophysical profile score.

CLINICAL SYMPTOMS: Decreased fetal movements.

BIOPHYSICAL PROFILE SCORE: FINDINGS: A single active intrauterine gestation is identified in longitudinal lie and cephalic presentation with AFI measured at 9.7 on today's exam. This places it within normal limits. Fetal heart rate is recorded at 115 beats/min. Fetus received scores of 2 for fetal breathing movements, fetal movements, fetal tone, and amniotic fluid volume for a total of 8 out of 8.

IMPRESSION
1. Biophysical profile score is 8 out of 8.
2. Fetal heart rate is recorded at 115 beats/min at both beginning and end of the exam. Clinical correlation is suggested.

CPT Code(s): _____

ICD-9-CM Code(s): _____

ICD-10-CM Code(s): _____

Abstracting Questions

1. Is this evaluation done with or without non-stress testing? _____

2. Why would decreased fetal movements be reported with a code from Category 655? _____

Case 83: Ultrasound, Abdominal

LOCATION: Outpatient, Hospital

PATIENT: Matt Rodriquez

PHYSICIAN: Morton Monson, MD

EXAMINATION OF: Abdominal ultrasound, RUQ.

CLINICAL SYMPTOMS: Right upper quadrant (RUQ) abdominal pain.

FINDINGS: This limited ultrasound to the gallbladder contains several small echogenic foci in the posterior aspect of the fundus, which do not appear to move but which do produce a small amount of shadowing. No gallbladder wall thickening, pericholecystic fluid, intrahepatic or extrahepatic ductal dilatation is identified with the common bile duct measuring 3 mm. Gallbladder is distended at 9 cm.

IMPRESSION
1. Distended gallbladder.
2. Small echogenic nonmobile foci in the fundus of the gallbladder. Differential considerations include adherent stones, polyps, or thrombus.

CPT Code(s): _____

ICD-9-CM Code(s): _____

ICD-10-CM Code(s): _____

Abstracting Questions

1. Is the ultrasound a complete or limited exam? _____

2. Was a definitive diagnosis determined? _____

Case 84: Computed Tomography, Groin

LOCATION: Outpatient, Hospital

PATIENT: Lindsay Reimer

PHYSICIAN: Morton Monson, MD

EXAMINATION OF: CT of right groin, including most of right femur.

CLINICAL SYMPTOMS: Infection vascular graft.

CT OF RIGHT GROIN, INCLUDING MOST OF RIGHT FEMUR: TECHNIQUE: Imaging from a level of the upper portion of the iliac crests through the distal right femoral shaft to the metadiaphyseal region using 7.5-mm collimation, table speed of 27, and pitch of 1.35 to 1 after oral contrast. There was IV contrast given for the chest CT, which preceded this study.

FINDINGS: Again seen is the comminuted fracture in the right hip region, which has been repaired. A significant amount of spray artifact is noted from the repair. There is soft tissue heterogeneous density about this area, which may represent hematoma. There is a vascular graft seen anteromedially about the groin and thigh, which appears to be seen in its proximal extent starting at image #17 and extending caudally to image #59. Along the proximal aspect of this graft, there is some stranding within the surrounding fat and increased density, which is similar to that surrounding the comminuted fracture of the hip. It is presumed that this is hematoma as this area was recently biopsied and negative cultures were obtained. The soft tissue and strandy density surrounding the proximal portion of the graft is noted only on levels where the fluid collections around the hip bony fragments are noted. Once you descend more caudally into the thigh, the fat around the graft demonstrates less strandiness and soft tissue density and is unremarkable in its appearance. There is some minimal diffuse bilateral subcutaneous strand-like density involving both upper thighs, although it is perhaps slightly more prominent on the right and in the lateral portion of the thigh away from the graft. The distal portion of the graft is unremarkable as well.

IMPRESSION: Fracture about the right hip, status post repair, with heterogeneous fluid surrounding the bony fragments, presumed to be due to hematoma, as this was recently biopsied and negative cultures were obtained. There is some strandlike density around the proximal portion of the graft at a similar level as the bony fracture fragments, but once you descend caudally into the lower portions of the thigh, that heterogeneous strandlike density is no longer visualized, and thus it is assumed that this strandlike density is made up of the same fluid as that surrounding the bony fragments about the hip. The mid and distal portions of the graft are essentially unremarkable.

CPT Code(s): _____

ICD-9-CM Code(s): _____

ICD-10-CM Code(s): _____

Abstracting Questions

1. Does the exam include contrast? _____

2. Is the complication evaluated as an infection of the graft? _____

Case 85: Computed Tomography, Chest

LOCATION: Outpatient, Hospital

PATIENT: Coby Leigh

PHYSICIAN: Morton Monson, MD

EXAMINATION OF: CT of chest.

CLINICAL SYMPTOMS
1. Shortness of breath.
2. Evaluate thoracic aortic short-segment graft just distal to subclavian takeoff of aorta, status post coronary bypass.

CT OF CHEST: TECHNIQUE: Imaging through the chest after 100 cc of iohexol 300 IV.

FINDINGS: The patient remains intubated. Small nodes are noted within the axilla. A tube is seen within the esophagus. Small lymph nodes are noted within the mediastinum, including pretracheal and precarinal areas. There is a small amount of pleural fluid on the right with presumed associated atelectasis. There is also pleural fluid on the left. There is some heterogeneous opacity, which appears to have some branching low-density areas within it, which is of uncertain etiology. Pneumonia or other etiology is possible. The adrenal glands are unremarkable. Diffuse emphysematous change with a large bulla is seen anteriorly within the right mid lung adjacent to the anterior junction line. The aorta is unremarkable. No definite evidence of a periaortic graft abscess is seen. However, this collection of pleural fluid and opacity with branching air density within it is identified.

IMPRESSION
1. Right pleural effusion with presumed atelectasis.
2. Left pleural effusion with increased associated opacity, which demonstrates a branching air pattern within it in the soft tissue windows. This may represent pneumonia. Other etiologies are possible but believed to be less likely.
3. No definite evidence of periaortic graft abscess.
4. Diffuse emphysematous change within the lungs with bullous change.

CPT Code(s): _____

ICD-9-CM Code(s): _____

ICD-10-CM Code(s): _____

Abstracting Questions

1. Is the CT done with contrast? _____

2. Is a more definitive diagnosis than shortness of breath determined? _____

3. Is the existence of the coronary artery bypass graft reported? _____

Case 86: Computed Tomography, Cranial

LOCATION: Outpatient, Hospital

PATIENT: Julius Vern

PHYSICIAN: Morton Monson, MD

EXAMINATION OF: Unenhanced cranial CT.

CLINICAL SYMPTOMS: Headache.

UNENHANCED CRANIAL CT: TECHNIQUE: Unenhanced axial images were acquired.

FINDINGS: Ventricles are normal in size and morphology. There is no intracranial hemorrhage or mass. Basal cisterns and falx are unremarkable. Mucosal thickening is noted at the dome of the right maxillary sinus. Mastoid air cells are clear.

IMPRESSION: Mucosal thickening at the dome of the visualized portions of the right maxillary sinus. The study is otherwise unremarkable.

CPT Code(s): _____

ICD-9-CM Code(s): _____

ICD-10-CM Code(s): _____

Abstracting Questions

1. Was contrast used for this exam? _____

2. Was there a more definitive diagnosis than presenting headache determined? _____

Case 87: Computed Tomography, Neck

LOCATION: Outpatient, Hospital

PATIENT: Scott Gail

PHYSICIAN: Morton Monson, MD

EXAMINATION OF: CT soft tissue neck.

CLINICAL SYMPTOMS: Right neck mass.

COMPUTED TOMOGRAPHIC EXAMINATION OF THE SOFT TISSUES OF THE NECK: Performed from the base of the skull to the superior mediastinum during rapid infusion of contrast material. The study was performed in my absence and is presented this morning for evaluation.

On the right, there is a prominent soft tissue structure (presumed enlarged lymph node) at the jugulodigastric junction (images 39 and 38). This measures approximately 15 mm in longest AP dimension (versus 10-11 mm on the left side). I do not appreciate other evidence of potential adenopathy. Fat planes are preserved. Airway is unremarkable.

IMPRESSION: Enlargement of single lymph node on the right as described above at the jugulodigastric junction. This might well be inflammatory, but histology cannot be predicted by a CT examination. This needs clinical correlation for the physical examination.

CPT Code(s): _____

ICD-9-CM Code(s): _____

ICD-10-CM Code(s): _____

Abstracting Questions

1. Was contrast used for this exam? _____

2. Was the reading physician present for the study? _____

3. Was there a definitive diagnosis other than the presenting problem? _____

4. Since "histology cannot be predicted by CT," what is likely the next step in the patient's treatment plan?

_____

5. What is meant by "clinical correlation"? _____

6. Does measurement of the mass affect code assignment? _____

Case 88: Computed Tomography, Neck

LOCATION: Outpatient, Hospital

PATIENT: Monica French

PHYSICIAN: Morton Monson, MD

EXAMINATION OF: CT of the soft tissues of the neck.

CLINICAL SYMPTOMS: Dysphagia, neck fullness.

COMPUTED TOMOGRAPHIC EXAMINATION OF THE SOFT TISSUES OF THE NECK:
Performed from the base of the skull to the superior mediastinum during rapid infusion of
contrast material. There is a small structure of slightly low density (compared with adjacent
musculature) in the midline at the hyoid bone. This is approximately 1 cm in AP dimension ×
6 to 7 mm in mediolateral dimension. Posterior fat plane of the preepiglottic space is normal.

I do not appreciate other abnormal soft tissue mass in the examination.

No adenopathy. Airway is unremarkable. Major vascular structures are well visualized with the
contrast infusion.

IMPRESSION: Small cystic structure in relation to the hyoid bone. I believe this is a
thyroglossal duct cyst. The remainder of the examination appears normal.

CPT Code(s): _____

ICD-9-CM Code(s): _____

ICD-10-CM Code(s): _____

Case 89: Computed Tomography, Sinusitis

LOCATION: Outpatient, Hospital

PATIENT: Joseph Stone

PHYSICIAN: Morton Monson, MD

EXAMINATION OF: CT of paranasal sinuses.

CLINICAL SYMPTOMS: Chronic sinusitis.

COMPUTED TOMOGRAPHIC EXAMINATION OF THE PARANASAL SINUSES: Performed in the coronal plane utilizing thin overlapping sections computed for high-resolution bone algorithm. Ultrathin (1-mm) sections were performed through the drainage pathways of the maxillary sinuses. Frontal sinuses are generous in size. They are well aerated. However, there is mucosal thickening inferiorly near the frontal nasal duct of each side.

Many ethmoid sinuses are clear and well aerated without significant mucosal abnormality. However, some ethmoid sinuses show mucosal thickening and several ethmoid sinuses show abnormal soft tissue within.

In images 20 and 21, there is a 1 cm in diameter soft tissue mass on the left. I believe this is within the ethmoid complex, rather than the left sphenoid sinus. I believe the sphenoid sinuses are clear and well aerated. Bilaterally, the maxillary sinuses are well aerated, but they both show considerable mucosal thickening and/or granulation tissue from previous inflammatory episodes. I cannot visualize a patent drainage pathway of either of the maxillary sinuses. I believe these are occluded. Nasal septum shows mild deviation to the right. Superior half of the nasal cavity is compromised of ethmoid air cells entering the middle turbinate. Some of the mucosal nodulations related to the ethmoid and maxillary sinuses have rounded margins and might represent polyps.

CPT Code(s): _____

ICD-9-CM Code(s): _____

ICD-10-CM Code(s): _____

Abstracting Questions

1. Was contrast material used? _____

2. Was there a more definitive diagnosis to report after examination? _____

3. Is the mild septal deviation reported? _____

Case 90: Magnetic Resonance Imaging, Forefoot

LOCATION: Outpatient, Hospital

PATIENT: Kimberly Adam

PHYSICIAN: Morton Monson, MD

EXAMINATION OF: MRI of left forefoot.

CLINICAL SYMPTOMS: Cellulitis.

MRI OF LEFT FOREFOOT: TECHNIQUE: T1 and fast spin-echo T2-weighted fat-saturation images of the left forefoot were obtained from the tarsometatarsal junction through the toes. Additional STIR coronal images were also obtained.

FINDINGS: There is extensive increased T2 signal present within the soft tissues of the left forefoot, consistent with edematous change. Findings are compatible with the clinical history of cellulitis. There is abnormal increased T2 signal present within the distal phalanx of the left great toe. A small amount of T1 abnormality is also seen in this area. Findings are compatible with osteomyelitis of the distal phalanx of the great toe. There is also some increased signal seen within the distal aspect of the proximal phalanx of the great toe, which is worrisome for additional osteomyelitis in this area. Increased T2 signal is seen within the third and possibly the second distal phalanx as well. This is near the edge of the coil and may be artifactual. The possibility of additional osteomyelitis of the second and third distal phalanges cannot be excluded. Close clinical correlation is suggested. The remainder of the marrow signal demonstrates some mild patchy increased T2 signal within the distal aspect of the midfoot. That is in a pattern, which we believe is most compatible with degenerative change.

IMPRESSION
1. Findings compatible with osteomyelitis of the distal phalanx of the left great toe, as well as the distal aspect of the proximal phalanx of the left great toe as well.
2. There is some apparent increased T2 signal seen within the second and third distal phalanges, which may be only technical; however, they could also relate to additional areas of osteomyelitis. Close clinical correlation is suggested.
3. Mildly increased T2 signal within the distal aspect of the midfoot is believed likely to be degenerative.
4. Prominent increased T2 signal is seen within the soft tissues of the left forefoot, in a pattern compatible with cellulitis.

CPT Code(s): _____

ICD-9-CM Code(s): _____

ICD-10-CM Code(s): _____

Abstracting Questions

1. Was contrast used? _____
2. Was examination of the foot tissues or the joints? _____
3. Does the location of the cellulitis affect diagnosis coding? _____
4. Is the osteomyelitis of the toes reported? _____

Case 91: Magnetic Resonance Imaging, Renal

LOCATION: Outpatient, Hospital

PATIENT: Jennifer Smith

PHYSICIAN: Morton Monson, MD

EXAMINATION OF: MRA of renal arteries.

CLINICAL SYMPTOMS: Hypertension, lupus, chronic renal failure.

MAGNETIC RESONANCE ANGIOGRAPHY OF THE RENAL ARTERIES: Performed in routine fashion with bolus injection following timing of the sequences with a test injection. For some reason, the venous vasculature (portal system and inferior vena cava) is also very prominent. Obviously, there was some error in timing. However, we have reviewed the procedure and cannot determine where the error might have occurred. I do certainly believe that the study is of diagnostic quality, particularly when viewed stereoscopically. I believe there is a single renal artery to each kidney. The initial several centimeters of each renal artery are visualized. I do not believe there is significant stenosis of either renal artery. Multiple vascular structures do show an intermittent string of beads appearance. This is artifactual. It does not represent fibromuscular dysplasia.

Abdominal aorta appears unremarkable.

IMPRESSION: For a technical reason that we have not been able to elucidate, venous structures are also prominently visualized, along with the arterial structures. I believe there is a single renal artery to each kidney. The initial several centimeters of each renal artery appear to be satisfactorily patent. The distal portions of the renal arteries and their branches cannot be evaluated. The abdominal aorta appears unremarkable. Because of the overlap of venous and arterial vasculature, stereoscopic viewing is very helpful. I have labeled the respective renal arteries on multiple images.

CPT Code(s): _____

ICD-9-CM Code(s): _____

ICD-10-CM Code(s): _____

Abstracting Questions

1. What anatomic region is listed in the index of the CPT? _____

2. If you search in the index of the CPT under Artery, Renal, Angiography, what codes are located and are they

   correct for this study? _____

3. What structure(s) was/were evaluated? _____

4. Is the code choice affected if the study is unilateral or bilateral? _____

5. Is the diagnosis for hypertension reported with renal involvement? _____

Case 92: Magnetic Resonance Imaging, Finger

LOCATION: Outpatient, Hospital

PATIENT: Bonnie Budge

PHYSICIAN: Morton Monson, MD

EXAMINATION OF: MR evaluation of left ring finger with recurrent episodes of cellulitis and lymphangitis.

MR EVALUATION OF LEFT RING FINGER: There are plain films of ring finger. Those show some deformity and a relatively thinned appearance to the shaft of the distal phalanx of the left ring finger. It is mainly deformity involving the medial aspect of the shaft of the distal phalanx of the left ring finger.

The AP dimension is normal. No cortical loss or destructive change is seen, and no soft tissue swelling is noted. Multiple MR sequences in sagittal, coronal, and axial projections are performed. There is no evidence of ongoing cellulitis of the left ring finger. There is no edema of the subcutaneous tissue or skin. There is no abnormal signal within the bone or bone marrow to suggest infection of bone or bone marrow. There is no circumscribed tumor or mass. Bony remodeling of the distal phalanx is likely due to multiple past episodes of inflammation. There is no current suggestion of mass in the left finger or abscess in the left finger.

IMPRESSION
1. No sign of inflammation of soft tissues or bone or bone marrow at present time. Imaged portions of left ring finger are unremarkable.
2. The bony deformity of the shaft of the distal phalanx that was seen on plain film of 07/13/XX is therefore believed to be old, due to remote injury or trauma.
3. No mass lesion seen currently.
4. No abscess identified.
5. No evidence of cellulitis or osteomyelitis involving left ring finger.

CPT Code(s): _____

ICD-9-CM Code(s): _____

ICD-10-CM Code(s): _____

Abstracting Questions

---

1. Would the cellulitis be reported? _____

Case 93: Magnetic Resonance Imaging, Brain

LOCATION: Outpatient, Hospital

PATIENT: Chad Allen

PHYSICIAN: Morton Monson, MD

EXAMINATION OF: MRI of brain.

CLINICAL SYMPTOMS: Slurred speech, right arm weakness.

MAGNETIC RESONANCE EXAMINATION OF THE BRAIN: Performed utilizing
T1-weighted sagittal views as well as spin density and T2-weighted sequences in the axial plane.
These were supplemented with axial T1-weighted sequence following intravenous infusion of
paramagnetic contrast material. Diffusion sequence was also performed.

In the spin density and T2-weighted sequences (images 17 and 18 of series 3), there is a small,
localized area of occipital cortex that shows increased intensity. This is also bright in the
diffusion sequence. This area is not hyperintense in the ADC map.

I do not appreciate significant abnormal increased or decreased intensity within brain
parenchyma of the remainder of the supratentorial brain. However, there is bilateral, irregularly
shaped, increased intensity within the pontine tegmentum. This is not hyperintense in the
diffusion sequence.

Ventricles are of normal size. Normal gray-white matter delineation is present. No abnormal
contrast enhancement of brain parenchyma.

IMPRESSION: Small hyperintense area of the cortex of the right occipital lobe, as described
above. This is also hyperintense in the diffusion sequence, but not in the ADC map. This would
indicate that this represents limited subacute infarction. I do not appreciate other areas of
subacute infarction. Remainder of supratentorial portion of the brain is unremarkable. The
pontine tegmentum is hazy with increased intensity within. This is not unusual in the older age
group (eighth and ninth decades of life), and is sometimes thought to represent evidence of
microvascular ischemic change. However, it is rarely indeterminate. In this case, I do not
appreciate evidence of enlargement of the brainstem, nor is there abnormal enhancement to
suggest neoplasm. I cannot elucidate further.

CPT Code(s): _____

ICD-9-CM Code(s): _____

ICD-10-CM Code(s): _____

Abstracting Questions

1. Is contrast used? _____

2. Were multiple sequences performed? _____

3. Does this affect code selection? _____

4. Do findings affect diagnostic coding of presenting problems? _____

Case 94: Doppler Study, Arterial

LOCATION: Outpatient, Hospital

PATIENT: Samual Krieger

PHYSICIAN: Morton Monson, MD

The patient is a 70-year-old man with diabetes and claudication symptoms. He is also a smoker and has renal failure. He has an ulcer on the right third toe, which is not healing.

This limited bilateral study is markedly abnormal. The ankle brachial index is 0.33 in the right and 0.47 on the left. Digital pressures are 0 on both sides. The "waveforms" are abnormal throughout both legs, indicating a "proximal level of occlusion in both legs," which is really quite severe. It appears that he does not have adequate circulation for healing at this time.

CONCLUSIONS: Severe bilateral arterial insufficiency, proximal in location.

CPT Code(s): _____

ICD-9-CM Code(s): _____

ICD-10-CM Code(s): _____

Abstracting Questions

1. What body area arteries are studied? _____

2. Is a definitive diagnosis determined? _____

Case 95: X-Ray, Chest

LOCATION: Outpatient, Hospital

PATIENT: Jim Fredricks

PHYSICIAN: Morton Monson, MD

EXAMINATION OF: Chest.

CLINICAL SYMPTOMS: Aortic aneurysm.

PORTABLE AP CHEST: FINDINGS: Comparison is made with the portable AP chest of 09/16/XX. Sternotomy. The right internal jugular catheter is seen, with tip in the upper superior vena cava. There is subsegmental atelectasis in the right infrahilar region. The left lung is clear. No pleural effusions. Borderline cardiac enlargement is unchanged. Pulmonary vascularity is likely within normal limits.

CPT Code(s): _____

ICD-9-CM Code(s): _____

ICD-10-CM Code(s): _____

Abstracting Questions

1. How many views were done? _____

2. What was that view projection? _____

3. Do the findings change the diagnosis of the presenting problem? _____

Case 96: X-Ray, Video Pharyngogram

LOCATION: Outpatient, Hospital

PATIENT: April Townsgard

PHYSICIAN: Morton Monson, MD

EXAMINATION OF: Video pharyngogram.

CLINICAL SYMPTOMS: Dysphagia.

VIDEO PHARYNGOGRAM: FINDINGS: A video pharyngogram was performed in conjunction with speech pathology. The patient was evaluated with $^1/_2$ tsp of puree and $^1/_2$ tsp of honey-thickened barium liquid. Both of the patient's swallows were very ineffective with a significant accumulation of contrast in the area of the valleculae and piriform sinuses. The patient did demonstrate aspiration on both of the consistencies. No additional evaluation was performed.

CPT Code(s): _____

ICD-9-CM Code(s): _____

ICD-10-CM Code(s): _____

Abstracting Questions

1. Does the swallow study affect the code reported? _____

2. Do the findings change the reported diagnosis? _____

Case 97: X-Ray, Abdomen

LOCATION: Outpatient, Hospital

PATIENT: Jon Mack

PHYSICIAN: Morton Monson, MD

EXAMINATION OF: Abdomen.

CLINICAL SYMPTOMS: Abdominal pain.

FLAT UPRIGHT ABDOMEN: FINDINGS: No comparison films are available.

On the upright portion of the exam, no free air is identified beneath the diaphragm. The study is somewhat limited by patient's body habitus.

On the upright portion of the exam, no differential air-fluid levels are visualized. Scattered small and large bowel gas is present. No small bowel dilatation is identified. On the flat plate, there is mild prominence to colon in the right upper quadrant, but this has a more normal appearance on the upright portion of the exam. There is extensive fecal material seen in the colon. No definite gas is identified in the region of the rectum, but study is somewhat limited by patient's habitus on the upright portion. Gas is seen in the region of the stomach and gas is seen in the region of the descending colon.

IMPRESSION: Nonspecific bowel gas pattern without evidence of obstruction. Follow up as clinically indicated.

CPT Code(s): _____

ICD-9-CM Code(s): _____

ICD-10-CM Code(s): _____

Abstracting Questions

1. How many views were taken? _____

2. Is there a definitive diagnosis to report as a finding? _____

Chapter 11
Interventional Radiology, Radiation Oncology, and Nuclear Medicine

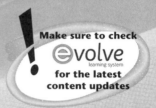
Make sure to check
evolve
learning system
for the latest
content updates

Case 98: Aspiration and Biopsy, Right Hip

LOCATION: Outpatient, Hospital

PATIENT: Tim Spears

INTERVENTIONAL RADIOLOGIST: Edward Riddle, MD

EXAMINATION OF: Aspiration and biopsy of inflammatory tissue of the right hip.

CLINICAL SYMPTOMS: Chronically dislocated right hip.

ASPIRATION AND BIOPSY OF INFLAMMATORY TISSUE OF THE RIGHT HIP: Patient has numerous medical problems. He is known to have a chronically dislocated right hip. One of his medical problems is consistent culturing of bacteria from the blood. Recent CT examination of the abdominal pelvic region showed inflammatory-thickened tissue in relation to the right hip region. There was question of infection at that site.

Unfortunately, we cannot use contrast material because of the patient's renal failure. Therefore, one cannot be certain if there are areas of necrosis and/or pus formation. I chose an area within this inflammatory mass that appeared to be of somewhat decreased density compared with the surrounding tissues. Appropriate access was determined using CT guidance, and the skin was marked, prepped, draped, and anesthetized. A 19-gauge, angiographic sheath was positioned into the area, which I believed showed low density. I could not aspirate pus. Two core biopsies were then obtained with an 18-gauge Cook unit. These were sent for appropriate cultures and Gram stain. The procedure was then terminated. The patient was returned to heparin. Official microbiologic results are awaited.

Pathology Report Later Indicated: Normal cultures. Inflamed subcutaneous tissue specimen.

CPT Code(s): _____

ICD-9-CM Code(s): _____

ICD-10-CM Code(s): _____

Abstracting Questions

1. What procedures are reported? _____

2. Was the biopsy of bone or muscle? _____

3. Was the biopsy superficial, deep, or percutaneous? _____

4. Is there a parenthetical note regarding imaging guidance with the biopsy code? _____

5. Is there a definitive diagnosis to report? _____

6. Is the chronic hip dislocation reported? _____

Case 99: Insertion Peripheral Catheter

OPERATIVE REPORT

LOCATION: Outpatient, Hospital

PATIENT: Michelle Kitty

PREOPERATIVE DIAGNOSIS: Necrotic skin of right foot.

POSTOPERATIVE DIAGNOSIS: Same.

INTERVENTIONAL RADIOLOGIST: Edward Riddle, MD

PROCEDURE PERFORMED: Insertion of central venous peripheral catheter.

INDICATION: Vascular access for long-term IV antibiotics.

PROCEDURE: The 65-year-old patient was informed of the risks and benefits prior to the procedure, and the consent was signed. The patient understands the risks and benefits and does accept. The right cephalic and right median cubital veins were identified and cleansed with 70% isopropyl alcohol and 2% chlorhexidine gluconate. The area was then allowed to dry for 30 seconds. A tourniquet was then applied. A 17-gauge introducer was unsuccessfully placed × one to the right cephalic and × one to the right median. The left median cubital vein was cleansed with 70% isopropyl alcohol and 2% chlorhexidine gluconate. The area was then allowed to dry for 30 seconds. A sterile drape was applied in the usual fashion. A tourniquet was then applied.

A 22-gauge IV catheter was placed. Good flow of blood was documented.

Subsequently, a guidewire was placed. The 22-gauge IV catheter was removed. A small incision was made to facilitate the introducer and dilator, which were placed successfully. The dilator was removed and a silicone Per-Q-Cath catheter was placed without difficulty up to 56 cm. There was return of blood flow after the guidewire was removed. It was flushed with normal saline, followed by heparin. The area was then dressed. A postprocedure chest x-ray has been obtained, checking for line placement.

CPT Code(s): _____

ICD-9-CM Code(s): _____

ICD-10-CM Code(s): _____

Abstracting Questions

1. Does the age of the patient affect catheter code reported? _____

2. Is there a pump or port? _____

3. Was imaging guidance used for line placement? _____

4. Is the postprocedure chest x-ray reported? _____

5. What diagnosis is used to report this service? _____

Case 100: Tunneled Catheter

OPERATIVE REPORT

LOCATION: Outpatient, Hospital

PATIENT: Matt Dilan

INTERVENTIONAL RADIOLOGIST: Edward Riddle, MD

EXAMINATION OF: Right IJV tunneled catheter placement.

CLINICAL SYMPTOMS: Chronic renal failure; dialysis access required.

RIGHT IJV TUNNELED DIALYSIS CATHETER PLACEMENT: This procedure is performed on a 48-year-old male. Informed consent was obtained. The right neck and clavicular region were prepped and draped in the usual sterile fashion. Skin and subcutaneous tissues were infiltrated with 1% lidocaine. Under ultrasound guidance, access was obtained into the right external jugular vein (EJV) and over a 0.035 three-tip guidewire. The needle was removed. Skin and subcutaneous tissues were sequentially dilated, followed by placement of a 15 French peel-away sheath. A subcutaneous tunnel was created from the right infraclavicular region to the right EJV puncture site. A 14.5 French Bard Hemosplit catheter was placed through the tunnel and then through the peel-away sheath. The sheath was removed. Under fluoroscopic observation, the distal tip of the dialysis catheter was placed in the right atrium. The catheter was secured to the skin with 2–0 Ethilon. The right neck incision was closed using vertical mattress suture technique with 3–0 Ethilon suture.

The patient received conscious sedation. The patient's pulse oximeter and vital signs were monitored throughout the exam. There were no complications. The patient tolerated the procedure well and left the radiology department in stable condition.

A single digital spot radiograph obtained demonstrates placement of the 14.5 French tunneled dialysis catheter via a right EJV approach with the distal tip of the catheter in the right atrium.

IMPRESSION: Successful and uncomplicated placement of a 14.5 French Bard Hemosplit catheter via a right EJV approach with the distal tip of the catheter in the right atrium.

CPT Code(s): _____

ICD-9-CM Code(s): _____

ICD-10-CM Code(s): _____

Case 101: Radiation Oncology Treatment Planning

LOCATION: Outpatient, Hospital

PATIENT: Tammy Parton

PHYSICIAN: James Eagle, MD

DIAGNOSIS: Stage II (T1cN1M0) grade 2 infiltrating ductal carcinoma involving the upper inner quadrant of the left breast. She underwent a partial segmentectomy with axillary node dissection with histopathology confirming a grade 2 cancer with two positive axillary lymph nodes. She has completed a course of systemic chemotherapy and now presents for consideration of adjuvant postoperative radiation.

CLINICAL CONSIDERATIONS: This patient is a 53-year-old female with a stage II carcinoma of the left breast. She does have several high-risk factors for local regional recurrence, which include grade, size, and positive lymph nodes. The indication, goals, and side effects of adjuvant postoperative radiotherapy to the chest wall and supraclavicular region have been discussed in detail. The patient appears to understand and has verbalized her desire to proceed with this option.

TECHNICAL CONSIDERATIONS: The initial target volume will include the left breast and left supraclavicular region to be treated for a total of 28 fractions. A radiotherapy boost will then be delivered to the chest wall for an additional five fractions. Normal tissues, which need to be considered, include the ribs, pulmonary parenchymal tissue, brachial plexus, heart, and left humeral head.

The dose fractionation to the left breast and left supraclavicular region is 50.4 Gy in 28 fractions. We anticipate delivering a radiotherapy boost for an additional 10 Gy in five fractions using electrons with en face radiation field.

The radiotherapy treatment is technically complex. Since this case is curative, we do wish to avoid excessive morbidity. Therefore, careful treatment planning is required, which implies that a planning CT scan, 3D simulation, and a 3D treatment computer plan are indicated and will be performed. She will initiate her radiotherapy thereafter. All questions and concerns have been addressed.

CPT Code(s): _____

ICD-9-CM Code(s): _____

ICD-10-CM Code(s): _____

Abstracting Questions

1. What level of treatment planning is provided? _____

2. What is the primary reason for the treatment? _____

3. Is the specific location known for the primary site? _____

4. Is there a secondary location being considered? _____

5. Is the specific location known for the secondary site? _____

Case 102: Radiation Oncology 3D Simulation

LOCATION: Outpatient, Hospital

PATIENT: Sarah Patterson

PHYSICIAN: James Eagle, MD

DIAGNOSIS: Stage II (T1cN1M0) infiltrating ductal carcinoma involving the upper inner quadrant of the left breast. She has undergone a partial segmentectomy with axillary node dissection with histopathology demonstrating grade 2 infiltrating ductal carcinoma with two positive axillary lymph nodes with positive estrogen and progesterone receptors. She has completed her systemic chemotherapy and has elected to proceed with adjuvant postoperative radiotherapy for her breast cancer.

SIMULATION: After explaining the purpose of the simulation and procedure, she was placed on the simulation table in the supine position. Both arms were elevated above her head and immobilized with the use of a wing board. A planning CT scan was then obtained. Two isocenters were placed for the radiation treatment fields. The patient was then marked so that the treatment position could be reproduced on a daily basis.

The left breast and left lung were contoured. The CT data was transferred to the CMS 3D treatment computer. The radiation treatment fields for the left breast were established using opposing tangential radiation portals at 100 SAD. An additional radiation portal was set for the left supraclavicular region using an AP technique treated to a depth of 3 cm. Consideration will be given to using the posterior axillary boost if indicated. We anticipate using 6 MV photons for all fields, which will be customized with the use of multileaf collimators. The tangential fields to the chest wall will be augmented with the use of wedges. Dose calculations and a complex 3D treatment computer plan will be generated to optimize the delivered dose.

The treatment computer will determine the appropriate electron energy for the radiotherapy boost to the chest wall. A custom-made Cerrobend block will be designed for the electron field. Dose calculations will be performed to ensure the prescribed dose will be delivered to the target volume.

The entire simulation took 60 minutes. The patient tolerated the procedure very well and was discharged in stable condition. She will initiate her adjuvant postoperative radiotherapy next week.

CPT Code(s): _____

ICD-9-CM Code(s): _____

ICD-10-CM Code(s): _____

Abstracting Questions

1. What level of simulation is provided based on the definitions in the CPT? _____

Case 103: Brachytherapy

LOCATION: Outpatient, Hospital

PATIENT: Kevin Green

PREOPERATIVE DIAGNOSIS: Atherosclerotic heart disease that has undergone a coronary artery bypass graft with placement of a stent within the vein graft of the right coronary artery, which was found to be totally occluded per angiogram. He has just completed his angioplasty to the RCA (right coronary artery) to ensure a stent patency.

POSTOPERATIVE DIAGNOSIS: Same.

PHYSICIAN: James Eagle, MD

PROCEDURE PERFORMED: Coronary artery brachytherapy.

PROCEDURE: Following the angioplasty, the coronary artery brachytherapy catheter was inserted. Fluoroscopy was performed to ensure that the distal end of the brachytherapy catheter was located distal to the previously dilated intraluminal stenosis. It was believed that the total injured length was approximately 42 mm, and therefore would require a catheter length of 52 mm. The treatment diameter would also require catheter with a diameter of 3.5 mm. Accordingly, it was believed that the appropriate cardiac catheter required for the treatment was a diameter of 3.5 mm with an active length of 52 mm to deliver the prescribed dose of 20 Gy. The treatment time was 361 seconds. The coronary artery brachytherapy treatment was delivered without difficulty. The coronary artery brachytherapy catheter was then removed without incident. His respiratory rate, heart rate, and heart monitor were stable throughout the procedure.

The patient tolerated the procedure very well. He was transported to the cardiology holding room in stable condition.

CPT Code(s): _____

ICD-9-CM Code(s): _____

ICD-10-CM Code(s): _____

Abstracting Questions

1. What type was delivered—radioelement solution, intracavity, interstitial, remote afterloading?

   _____

2. How many catheters were placed for treatment? _____

3. Is the fluoroscopy also reported? _____

4. What was the diagnosis for which treatment was rendered? _____

5. Was the location of the occlusion specified? _____

Case 104: Myocardial Perfusion Scan

LOCATION: Outpatient, Hospital

PATIENT: Brock Blakley

PHYSICIAN: Morton Monson, MD

EXAMINATION OF: Stress and rest myocardial perfusion scan.

CLINICAL SYMPTOMS: Shortness of breath; pacemaker.

STRESS AND REST MYOCARDIAL PERFUSION SCAN: TECHNIQUE: A total of 29.5 millicuries of technetium-99m tetrofosmin was administered following stress with adenosine, and 26.5 millicuries of technetium-99m tetrofosmin was administered at rest. SPECT imaging was performed in all three planes.

FINDINGS: Ejection fraction is prominently decreased at 12%. On the previous study, it was 21%. On the static images used to calculate ejection fraction, there appears to be dyskinesis of the cardiac apex, the inferior wall, and portions of the lateral wall.

There is dilatation of the cardiac chamber. Decreased myocardial perfusion is seen in the inferior wall, with only minimal reversibility. Decreased myocardial perfusion in the cardiac apex extends into the periapical anterior wall, and this is a mixed myocardial perfusion defect, with some reversibility. There is thinning of the lateral wall and septum, but these are not significantly reversible on rest images, and the septum actually appears somewhat worsened on rest images.

IMPRESSION:
1. Predominantly fixed myocardial perfusion defect involves the inferior wall, though there is minimal reversibility.
2. Mixed myocardial perfusion defect involving the cardiac apex and periapical anteroseptum.
3. Mild thinning of the lateral wall and more prominently the septum, which is not reversible.
4. Dilatation of the cardiac chamber.
5. Prominently decreased ejection fraction at 12%. Please see above comments.

CPT Code(s): _____

ICD-9-CM Code(s): _____

ICD-10-CM Code(s): _____

Abstracting Questions

1. Was the study done at rest, stress, or both? _____

2. Was a single study or multiple studies done? _____

3. Was SPECT utilized? _____

Case 105: Nuclear Stress Test

LOCATION: Outpatient, Hospital

PATIENT: Opal Hanson

PHYSICIAN: Morton Monson, MD

EXAMINATION OF: Stress test.

CLINICAL SYMPTOMS: Chest pain.

STRESS TEST: TECHNIQUE: The patient received adenosine under the supervision of Dr. Marvin Elhart. The patient also received 30.2 millicuries of Tc-99m tetrofosmin for the stress portion of the study.

The patient received 23.9 millicuries of Tc-99m tetrofosmin for the resting portion of the study. Stress and rest SPECT images of the left ventricle were obtained.

FINDING: Reversible perfusion defects, involving the posterior/inferior wall extending somewhat into the cardiac apex and lateral wall. Mild thinning of the anteroseptal wall could be artifactual. The calculated ejection fraction is 53%, normal being 50% or greater.

CPT Code(s): _____

ICD-9-CM Code(s): _____

ICD-10-CM Code(s): _____

Chapter 12
Cardiology

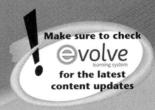

Make sure to check
evolve
learning system
**for the latest
content updates**

Case 106: Cardioversion

LOCATION: Outpatient, Hospital

PATIENT: Madison Flare

PHYSICIAN: James Nooner, MD

PROCEDURE PERFORMED: Cardioversion.

PROCEDURE: The patient was sedated. Under cardiac monitoring and pulse oximetry monitoring, the patient received 360 joules of synchronous energy with successful cardioversion to sinus rhythm.

IMPRESSION: Successful cardioversion from atrial fibrillation to sinus rhythm. The patient will be started on sotalol.

CPT Code(s): _____

ICD-9-CM Code(s): _____

ICD-10-CM Code(s): _____

Abstracting Questions

1. Was this an external or internal cardioversion? _____
2. What was the presenting problem, and was it resolved? _____

Case 107: Pharmacologic Nuclear Perfusion Stress Test

LOCATION: Outpatient, Hospital

PATIENT: Jack Rider

PHYSICIAN: Marvin Elhart, MD

INDICATION: History of myocardial infarction 6 years ago, status post PTCA with stent 6 years ago, no further cardiovascular events.

CURRENT MEDICATIONS: Loratadine, Nephrocaps, digoxin, sertraline, albuterol, terazosin, morphine, glipizide, ranitidine, felodipine, quinine, sulfate, metoprolol, and furosemide.

The patient is 5'7" and 198 pounds.

PROCEDURE PERFORMED: Pharmacologic nuclear perfusion stress test.

PROCEDURE: After informed consent was obtained and the risks and benefits were explained, the patient was brought to the Cardiopulmonary Stress Lab and was outfitted with IV access for fluid administration of Persantine and Myoview, as well as continuous 12-lead electrocardiographic monitoring.

The patient received infusion of Persantine via peripheral IV access, a total of 45.3 mgm over a 4-minute interval in a volume of 9.1 cc. Initial heart rate was 69 beats/min, which reached a nadir of 61 beats/min throughout the pharmacologic portion of the study. Initial blood pressure was 167/85. It reached a nadir of 128/54 during the pharmacologic portion of the study. At 7 minutes, the patient received 30 millicuries of Myoview nuclear perfusion tracer agent injected as a bolus. At 10 minutes, the patient received 100 mgm of IV aminophylline as a bolus. Throughout the examination, the patient offered no complaints of chest pain, shortness of breath, palpitations, paresthesia, diaphoresis, claudication, light-headedness, or dizziness. No EKG change in the way of ventricular or supraventricular tachycardia; no ST changes, elevation with injury, or ST depression with ischemia; no P-R prolongation, AV block, or bundle branch block formation generated.

NUCLEAR PERFUSION IMAGING TO FOLLOW.

CONCLUSIONS
1. Functional capacity not assessed.
2. Double product.
3. Nuclear perfusion stress test with pharmacologic stressor agent performed using Persantine as a peripheral vasodilator 45.3 mgm and a volume of 9.1 cc over a 4-minute interval.
4. Initial heart rate 69 beats/min reached a nadir of 61 beats/min during the examination.
5. Initial blood pressure was 167/85 reached a nadir of 128/54 throughout the examination.
6. Appropriate heart rate and blood pressure response to pharmacologic stressor agent of Persantine.
7. Total number of METS 1.
8. Pharmacologic portion of the stress test discontinued once maximum vasodilation hyperemic effect achieved.
9. At 7 minutes, the patient received 30 millicuries of Myoview tetrofosmin base technetium perfusion tracer agent.
10. At 10-minute interval, the patient received 100 mgm of aminophylline IV push to complete the study.

11. Throughout the entire examination, the patient offered no complaints of chest pain, shortness of breath, palpitations, paresthesia, diaphoresis, claudication, light-headedness, or dizziness.

12. No EKG changes indicative of current of injury or ST depression or ischemia. No ectopy. No supraventricular or ventricular arrhythmia. No P-R prolongation, AV block, or bundle branch block formation.

13. Nuclear perfusion images to follow.

IMPRESSION: Equivocal pharmacologic portion of stress test with no EKG changes and no clinical signs or symptoms of ischemia or angina pectoris.

CPT Code(s): _____

ICD-9-CM Code(s): _____

ICD-10-CM Code(s): _____

Abstracting Questions

1. Does the use of medication versus patient testing on a treadmill or bicycle affect the code range?

   _____

2. Was this a total component reporting? _____

Case 108: Echocardiogram

LOCATION: Outpatient, Hospital

PATIENT: Edward Smart

PHYSICIAN: James Nooner, MD

REASON FOR TEST: Congestive heart failure.

Technically difficult study, only limited views available. Picture quality is poor. The following points were noted:
1. Overall left ventricular ejection fraction is diminished around 40% to 45%. It appears that the distal septum is hypokinetic. However, no definite comments can be passed on. There are some wall motion abnormalities due to technical difficulties.
2. Right ventricular function appears to be normal.
3. No significant pericardial effusion.
4. Aortic root and valve sclerosis with no significant restriction to the opening of the aortic valve. There is no significant aortic regurgitation.
5. Mitral annular calcification. Mitral valve is thickened. There is some restriction to the opening of the mitral valve, but no significant stenosis. There appears to be trace to mild mitral regurgitation.
6. Mitral inflow velocities reveal E to A reversal suggestive of impaired relaxation of the left ventricle. For exact quantification of ejection fraction, one may need to do a MUGA scan.

CPT Code(s): _____

ICD-9-CM Code(s): _____

ICD-10-CM Code(s): _____

Abstracting Questions

1. Was this a complete or limited exam? _____

2. Was the blood flow (movement of heart valves and ventricles) evaluated in this exam? _____

3. Was velocity of blood flow evaluated? _____

4. Is there a definitive diagnosis? _____

Case 109: Adenosine Myoview Stress Test

LOCATION: Outpatient, Hospital

PATIENT: Tiffany Otterson

PHYSICIAN: James Nooner, MD

INDICATIONS: Atherosclerotic heart disease.

Adenosine stress test was performed according to our routine protocol. The heart rate did not change significantly throughout the test.

The patient complained of stomach pressure that was relieved spontaneously.

There was no significant arrhythmia.

The underlying rhythm was 100% paced rhythm.

CONCLUSION
1. Nondiagnostic adenosine stress test for ischemia by electrocardiographic criteria.
2. Myoview results to follow.

CPT Code(s): _____

ICD-9-CM Code(s): _____

ICD-10-CM Code(s): _____

Case 110: Stress Test

LOCATION: Outpatient, Hospital

PATIENT: Jerry Rosengram

PHYSICIAN: Marvin Elhart, MD

INDICATIONS: The patient is status post myocardial infarction 6 months ago, CABG, and pacemaker.

This is a 70-year-old male, 5'8" and 170 pounds. On Epogen, Protonix, vancomycin, Plavix, insulin, and Colace. The patient underwent an adenosine stress test with Myoview injection.

HEMODYNAMIC RESPONSE: Heart rate at rest 76, at peak is 82. Blood pressure at rest at peak is 105/60. During the infusion of adenosine the patient had no complaints. He had a burning feeling. At baseline the patient had pacemaker rhythm that has not changed with the infusion.

CONCLUSION
1. Good vasodilator response to adenosine.
2. This EKG stress test is inconclusive for evidence of obstructive disease.
3. The Myoview part of the stress test will be reported separately.

CPT Code(s): _____

ICD-9-CM Code(s): _____

ICD-10-CM Code(s): _____

Case 111: Cardiac Catheterization Report

LOCATION: Outpatient, Hospital

PATIENT: Raymond Severson

PHYSICIAN: James Nooner, MD

PROCEDURE PERFORMED: Bilateral heart catheterization.

BRIEF HISTORY: This is a 52-year-old patient with known dilated cardiomyopathy with atherosclerotic heart disease. Increased shortness of breath was noted recently. Stress revealed dilated ventricle with depressed ejection fraction and inferior wall ischemia. Angiography was recommended. Bilateral heart catheterization was advised along with that. The patient understands the procedure, the indications, the alternatives and all of the potential complications, and agrees and consents for it. He consents for angioplasty and possible emergency bypass surgery.

PROCEDURE: The patient was brought to the Cath Lab. He was placed on the cath table, prepped, and draped in the usual fashion. The procedure was performed through the right femoral vessels using a 6 French arterial system and an 8 French venous system. At the end, the Perclose device was deployed without difficulty.

COMPLICATIONS: None.

FINDINGS:
I.   HEMODYNAMICS: Right atrial mean 7. RV 37/EDP 4. PA pressure 37/12 with mean of 21. Pulmonary wedge pressure 19/13 with mean of 13. LVEDP 20, LV pressure 162, aortic pressure 162/65 with mean of 98. Cardiac output 5.65 liters/min via thermodilution.

II. LEFT VENTRICULOGRAPHY: This was performed in the RAO projection. This revealed moderate to severe left ventricular enlargement. The overall left ventricular systolic function was severely depressed, estimated at 25%. There was asynchronous movement of the anterior wall. The base and inferior wall were dyskinetic. There was mild mitral insufficiency. No gradient across the aortic valve on pullback. There were diffuse coronary artery calcifications.

III. CORONARY ANGIOGRAPHY:
1. LEFT MAIN CORONARY ARTERY: Arises from the left coronary cusp. It has diffuse calcifications with mild luminal irregularities. No high-grade lesions.
2. LEFT ANTERIOR DESCENDING ARTERY: This is a diffusely diseased vessel that is rather slender. It gives rise to a very large high-rising diagonal that supplies a large area myocardium. This diagonal has mild luminal irregularities.
   This vessel, as a matter of fact, has a larger area of distribution than the LAD proper. After that, a second diagonal is seen to originate from the LAD that is slender and harbors 70% proximal stenosis. The LAD distal to that has diffuse luminal irregularities with tandem 40% to 50% stenoses.
3. LEFT CIRCUMFLEX ARTERY: Average size vessel that has a recurrent atrial branch. The circumference is diffusely diseased and has a long 50% stenosis in its mid segment. It terminates into a posterolateral that is diffusely diseased and culminates with an eccentric 30% to 40% stenosis.
4. RIGHT CORONARY ARTERY: Arises from the right coronary cusp. It is a very large vessel that is dominant in distribution. It has an eccentric 50% hazy stenosis proximally. Distally, it gives rise to a very large posterior descending artery that has two branches. The inferior

branch has tandem 70% stenosis distally. The right coronary artery has a terminal posterolateral that has an 80% localized stenosis.

5. SELECTIVE RIGHT ILIOFEMORAL INJECTION: Selective right iliofemoral injection reveals a widely patent vessel, suitable for Perclose, which was deployed without difficulty. This vessel has diffuse mild luminal irregularities.

CONCLUSION
1. Mild pulmonary hypertension with systemic hypertension.
2. Significant left ventricular dilation with severe LV dysfunction.
3. Diffuse coronary calcifications with atherosclerotic lesions.

IMPRESSION: The patient's LV dysfunction appears to be perhaps slightly worse than it was before. His coronary anatomy has not changed significantly. His lesions, even though some of them are tight, do not warrant revascularization. Clearly, this patient's cardiomyopathy is out of proportion to his ischemic heart disease, and I do suspect that alcoholic etiology has a significant portion to do with it.

PLAN: 1. Medical therapy. 2. Risk factor modification. 3. Coreg therapy. Because of the patient's bradycardia and left bundle branch block, he definitely will need to have a pacemaker implanted. I will evaluate this patient for the possibility of biventricular pacing with resynchronization therapy. The patient is in agreement to perform that, and I will have to make arrangements for that to be done.

CPT Code(s): _____

ICD-9-CM Code(s): _____

ICD-10-CM Code(s): _____

Abstracting Questions

1. What was the approach for the insertion of the catheter? _____

2. Is the imaging for the catheterization for the right heart, left heart, or both? _____

3. Are congenital anomalies or septal defects involved? _____

4. Is the imaging for the ventriculography reported in addition to the coronary angiography? _____

5. Are the injection procedures reported? _____

6. In addition to the cardiomyopathy and atherosclerotic heart disease, are the shortness of breath and abnormal stress test reported? _____

Case 112: Cardiac Catheterization Report

LOCATION: Outpatient, Hospital

PATIENT: Peter Noon

PHYSICIAN: Marvin Elhart, MD

BRIEF HISTORY: The patient is a 58-year-old gentleman with jaw pain and abnormal Cardiolite. Angiography was recommended to assess the presence or absence of ischemic heart disease. A radial approach was utilized as the patient had a normal Allen test. The patient understands the procedure with all the potential complications and agrees to proceed.

PROCEDURE: Left heart catheterization.

PROCEDURE NOTE: The patient was brought to the cardiac catheterization laboratory. His preprocedure labs were acceptable. He was placed on the cath table, prepped, and draped in the usual fashion. The procedure was performed through the right radial artery without complications.

FINDINGS
I. LEFT VENTRICULOGRAPHY: This was performed in the RAO projection. The LVEDP was 13. The LV pressure was 129. The aortic pressure was 129/73 with a mean of 96. Ejection fraction is estimated well above 55%.

There was no regional wall motion abnormality, mitral insufficiency, or gradient across the aortic valve on pullback.

II. CORONARY ANGIOGRAPHY:
1. LEFT MAIN CORONARY ARTERY: The left main coronary artery arises from the left coronary cusp. It is somewhat of a short vessel that is normal.
2. LEFT ANTERIOR DESCENDING ARTERY: This is an average size vessel that is tortuous with two average size diagonals. The LAD has minimal lumen irregularities proximally.
3. LEFT CIRCUMFLEX ARTERY: This is an average size vessel. It is a very tortuous obtuse marginal and somewhat of a tortuous terminal posterolateral, both of which appear to be free of significant disease.
4. RIGHT CORONARY ARTERY: The right coronary artery arises from the right coronary cusp. It is a large dominant vessel. It is larger than an average posterior descending artery and a posterolateral. There is no significant disease involving right coronary artery and its branches. There appears to be perhaps slight minimal luminal irregularities proximally.

CONCLUSION
1. Normal left ventricular systolic function.
2. Minimal insignificant atherosclerotic heart disease.

IMPRESSIONS AND PLANS
1. The patient's Cardiolite abnormality is false positive.
2. Jaw pain is noncardiac.
3. The patient should be treated aggressively for his hypertension and reassured. The patient will be discharged later on today.

CPT Code(s): _____

ICD-9-CM Code(s): _____

ICD-10-CM Code(s): _____

Chapter 13
Inpatient Cases

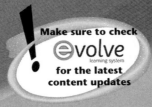

Make sure to check
evolve
learning system
**for the latest
content updates**

For these inpatient cases, assign all necessary diagnosis codes, E codes, V codes, and ICD-9-CM Volume 3 procedure codes.

Case 113: Fracture, Hip

There are three reports that are to be considered when coding this hospital stay.

ORTHOPEDIC ADMISSION HISTORY AND PHYSICAL

LOCATION: Inpatient, Hospital

PATIENT: Jamie Dale

ATTENDING PHYSICIAN: Mohomad Almaz, MD

CHIEF COMPLAINT: Left thigh pain.

PRESENT ILLNESS: The patient is a 50-year-old woman with chronic obstructive pulmonary disease (COPD) and is steroid dependent, on home oxygen. She apparently fell at home today when she tripped and twisted her left leg. She was seen in the emergency department, where x-rays revealed a supracondylar fracture of her left femur, and she was referred here because of this. On her arrival here, she was alert and cooperative. She complained of pain in her left leg just above her left knee, weightbearing increased the pain. Denies numbness and denies pain elsewhere. She told me that she normally was able to get around fairly well at home. She does have a long history of COPD. She is on prednisone 20 mg daily. According to some of the medical records that came with her, she has polycythemia vera. She apparently was a chronic smoker. She has severe pulmonary hypertension with congestive heart failure. She has had a cholecystectomy and appendectomy. She had a left humeral neck fracture in the past.

REVIEW OF SYSTEMS: Patient states she has had some weight loss and occasional dizziness.

PHYSICAL EXAMINATION: Today found that she is an alert and cooperative female, who arrived in the emergency department lying on a cart with the left leg in a long leg splint applied by the ambulance crew and secured with Velcro straps. She appeared to be fairly comfortable. She was able to easily answer questions, and she moved her upper extremities well and moved her right leg well. She appeared to be aware of her surroundings and oriented to place and time. Examination of her left leg found that the foot was externally rotated. She was, however, able to dorsiflex and plantar flex her foot and toes. The dorsalis pedis pulse was easily palpable. There were no lacerations or abrasions about the left thigh. She had pain just above her left knee with any movement of the leg, however.

X-rays of her left femur found that she does have a comminuted displaced supracondylar fracture. The knee is seen on these views and the joint spaces appear to be fairly well preserved, although there is some calcification along the medial side of her knee joint.

IMPRESSION
1. Comminuted displaced supracondylar fracture, left femur.
2. History of chronic obstructive pulmonary disease, steroid dependent, on home oxygen.
3. Severe primary pulmonary hypertension with congestive heart failure.
4. Status post cholecystectomy and appendectomy.
5. Secondary polycythemia.
6. Status post left humeral neck fracture.

RECOMMENDATIONS: I have thoroughly discussed this left femur problem with her. I have recommended an open reduction internal fixation using a supracondylar plate. I have discussed the risks involved with her in detail, as she is a rather poor surgical risk. She understands that there is certainly a chance for an infection and there is certainly a chance for a nonunion or a malunion. Thrombophlebitis is a possibility. She may have a stroke or a heart attack. It is possible that she may have difficulty getting off a respirator if she has a general anesthetic. We have discussed all these and other possible risks. She would like to go ahead with the surgery. Her questions have been answered and she understands that there are very significant risks involved with this. She will be taken directly to surgery.

OPERATIVE REPORT

LOCATION: Inpatient, Hospital

PATIENT: Jamie Dale

ATTENDING PHYSICIAN: Mohomad Almaz, MD

SURGEON: Mohomad Almaz, MD

PREOPERATIVE DIAGNOSIS: Comminuted supracondylar fracture, left distal femur.

POSTOPERATIVE DIAGNOSIS: Comminuted supracondylar fracture, left distal femur.

PROCEDURE PERFORMED: Open reduction internal fixation of supracondylar fracture, left distal femur.

ANESTHESIA: Spinal.

FINDINGS: The patient was found to have a markedly comminuted and displaced supracondylar fracture. This extended down to the condyles, but it did not appear to enter the intercondylar area. This was a markedly comminuted fracture and her bone is quite soft. We were able to assemble many of the fragments in a near anatomic position and hold this in place with a supracondylar plate. Not all of the fragments, however, could be assembled in an anatomic position, and there was a step-off along the medial side of the distal femur, which persisted despite our best efforts to reduce this more anatomically. However, we were able to obtain what we felt was a stable reduction.

DESCRIPTION OF PROCEDURE: While under a spinal anesthetic the patient's left leg was prepped with Betadine and draped in a sterile fashion. She was given vancomycin and gentamicin preoperatively. We then created an incision over the lateral aspect of the left distal thigh and curved it slightly anteriorly toward the lateral aspect of the patella. We then carried the dissection down through the subcutaneous tissue and incised the fascia. We proceeded along the lateral intramuscular septum to the femur and reflected the vastus lateralis anteriorly and medially. We were able to identify the fracture. She did bleed very freely. We eventually elected to apply a sterile tourniquet, which we inflated to 300 mm Hg, and the total tourniquet time ended up being about 68 minutes. She did receive 3 units of packed cells during the procedure.

We then thoroughly irrigated the area with saline; we tried to assemble some of the comminuted fragments and hold them with a cerclage wire. This allowed us to determine the actual length of the femur, but it was still difficult to get all of the pieces assembled. We were able to hold the femur out to length as we applied a supracondylar plate. This was a 10-hole 95-degree supracondylar plate. We drilled a guidewire from the lateral femoral condyle to the medial femoral condyle using the wire guide. We then reamed to a depth of 90 mm and inserted an 80-mm lag screw to which we attached the 10-hole supracondylar plate. We then attached the plate to the shaft using cortical screws and also a couple of cancellous screws distally. The resultant fixation appeared to be satisfactory. We were able to place the knee through a range of motion. There did not appear to be any movement of the fracture site. Certainly we were very careful with this since the bone is not strong. We tried to assemble several of the fragments of bone to fill in the gaps. We then thoroughly irrigated the area with saline and closed the fascia using 0 Vicryl. We closed the subcutaneous tissue using 2–0 Vicryl. We then closed the skin using staples. Before closing the skin, however, we did obtain an AP and lateral x-ray of the left distal femur. We found that the overall alignment was acceptable. Certainly there was a step-off along the medial side of the distal shaft, which we could appreciate intraoperatively, but we elected to accept this since it was very difficult to align this fracture. She had Xeroform dressings applied to the incision and an ACE wrap was used over the 4 × 4 dressings. We then applied a knee immobilizer to the left leg. She was then transported from the operating room in good condition with breathing spontaneous. The final sponge and needle counts were correct. She will be continued on vancomycin for 48 hours. We will place her in the SCCU overnight at least. The estimated blood loss was 2000 cc. She did have 3 units of red blood cells given to her.

DISCHARGE SUMMARY

LOCATION: Inpatient, Hospital

PATIENT: Jamie Dale

ATTENDING PHYSICIAN: Mohomad Almaz, MD

PRINCIPAL DIAGNOSIS: Comminuted, displaced, supracondylar left femur fracture.

ADDITIONAL DIAGNOSES
1. Chronic obstructive pulmonary disease, steroid dependent.
2. Anemia.

PRINCIPAL PROCEDURE: Open reduction and internal fixation of left distal femur.

ALLERGIES: Cefoxitin, reaction uncertain.

MEDICATIONS: Please see chart.

HISTORY: This patient entered the hospital with chief complaint of left thigh pain. This lady apparently was at home when she fell and injured her left leg. She was seen in the emergency room where x-rays revealed a supracondylar fracture of her left femur. She was then referred down for further care of this injury. Examination found that her left foot was externally rotated. She did have pain with any movement of her left knee. X-rays of her left femur found that she did have a comminuted, displaced supracondylar fracture. Discussion was held, and recommendation was made that she be taken to the operating room for an open reduction and internal fixation procedure to stabilize her left femur fracture. She agreed and wanted to go ahead with this. She was taken to the operating room where, under spinal anesthesia, an open reduction and internal fixation of supracondylar fracture, left distal femur was carried out. At the end of the procedure, sterile dressings were applied, and her left leg was placed into a knee immobilizer. She tolerated the procedure well.

Postoperatively, she remained afebrile; other vital signs remained normal as well. Dressings were changed at intervals with no signs of infection noted.

CPT Code(s): _____

ICD-9-CM Code(s): _____

ICD-10-CM Code(s): _____

Abstracting Questions

1. What is the primary reason for this admission? _____

2. What other medical conditions affected management of this patient? _____

3. Are E codes reported to describe how and where injury occurred? _____

4. Was the fracture repair open or closed; internal or external fixation? _____

5. What should be reported in addition to the surgical procedure? _____

6. Does the type of transfusion affect code reported? _____

Case 114: Arthroplasty

There are four reports that are to be considered when coding this hospital stay.

HISTORY AND PHYSICAL EXAM

LOCATION: Inpatient, Hospital

PATIENT: Dina Olson

ATTENDING PHYSICIAN: Laddie N. Noss, MD

DIAGNOSIS: Left hip injury.

HISTORY OF PRESENT ILLNESS/PURPOSE OF VISIT: The patient is a 58-year-old female with a left hip injury. She was walking at home in her house when she subsequently tripped, fell, and landed on her left hip. She did not strike her head. No other injuries. No loss of consciousness. She only complains of left hip pain. This pain is stated as a throbbing, constant pain that is 8 of 10 in severity. She denies any new paresthesias. She was brought to the emergency department, and I was subsequently consulted. She was admitted secondary to a left hip fracture. Overall, she denies any other complaints other than left hip fracture. She is a household ambulator with a walker. I know Ms. Olson in the fact that I previously had treated her secondary to a distal tibia fracture some time ago, which was treated conservatively with casting. She required a significant amount of time in regard to poor healing.

REVIEW OF SYSTEMS: Complete review of systems performed and negative.

PAST MEDICAL HISTORY: Positive for:
1. Chronic renal disease, end-stage renal disease with renal transplant in 1986 and has been on hemodialysis for the past year.
2. Diabetes mellitus.
3. History of herpes zoster.
4. Mechanical low back pain with chronic pain.
5. Hypertension.
6. Acute myelogenous leukemia.
7. Depression.

PAST SURGICAL HISTORY
1. Status post lumbar surgery times two.
2. Status post TAH/BSO.
3. Status post appendectomy.
4. Status post left eye surgery.
5. Status post AV fistula placement.

FAMILY HISTORY: Family history of chronic pain.

ALLERGIES: No known drug allergies.

MEDICATIONS
1. Tylenol.
2. Claritin.
3. Colace.
4. Cozaar.
5. Epogen.
6. Folic acid.

7. Hydroxyzine.
8. Imodium.
9. Humalog insulin.
10. Lantus insulin
11. Naprosyn.
12. Procardia.
13. Reglan.
14. Renagel.
15. Ritalin.
16. Sarna.
17. Thiamine.
18. Zoloft.

Of note, in regard to her medications, I did obtain these from her old records. She is not completely cognizant of all her medications.

PHYSICAL EXAMINATION: A 58-year-old female. She is awake, alert, and oriented. She is conversant. Vital signs per ER note, which was reviewed and overall grossly stable. Both upper extremities' ranges of motion are without significant pain or discomfort. Right lower extremity range of motion is also without pain. Her left hip is mildly externally rotated. She has pain with any type of motion. She has no evidence of open lesions. No significant knee, leg, or ankle tenderness today. Her right ankle range of motion is without pain. In regard to her left ankle, her pulses are palpable, +1. She is able to plantar flex and dorsiflex at the ankle. Has fairly good strength. In regard to sensation, she does have relatively intact sensation to light touch, but proprioception sensation is diminished, and she does have difficulty telling which toes I am touching when palpating her left lower extremity.

X-RAYS: X-rays are reviewed. X-rays reveal a displaced left intertrochanteric fracture. She does demonstrate fairly ectatic femoral canal that is widened. Her fracture again is displaced. No marked osteoarthritis.

IMPRESSION: Left displaced femoral neck fracture.

PLAN: I had a discussion with the patient regarding the findings. Unfortunately, her fracture is displaced. I was originally hoping that her fracture would be nondisplaced so we could get by with pinning, but again there is a displacement. Due to her history, she is at a high risk for avascular necrosis and really the only option is hip arthroplasty. The two options would be a bipolar hemiarthroplasty versus a total hip arthroplasty. I think due to the fact that she is ambulatory and with her other complications, I think the total hip arthroplasty would be her best option. The main disadvantage of this would be the risk for dislocation. I have discussed total hip arthroplasty with her. We likely will have to use a cemented stem due to her fairly poor bone quality and her history of dialysis and renal failure. Labs have been ordered. I have discussed the risks, benefits, and alternatives to surgery including in the risk for superficial versus deep infection, neurovascular injury, leg length discrepancy, aseptic loosening, superficial versus deep infection, wound problems, DVT, PE, need for revision, and death. She is fully aware of this. She would like to proceed with operative intervention. I did also discuss code status, and she would like to remain code status I. Otherwise, all questions were answered.

OPERATIVE REPORT

LOCATION: Inpatient, Hospital

PATIENT: Dina Olson

ATTENDING PHYSICIAN: Laddie N. Noss, MD

SURGEON: Mohomad Almaz, MD

PREOPERATIVE DIAGNOSIS: Left displaced intertrochanteric fracture.

POSTOPERATIVE DIAGNOSIS: Same.

INDICATION: Relieve pain, restore function.

PROCEDURE: Left hip bipolar hemiarthroplasty.

ANESTHESIA: Spinal anesthesia.

ESTIMATED BLOOD LOSS: 200 cc.

COMPLICATIONS: None known.

HISTORY: The patient is a 58-year-old female who sustained a left displaced intertrochanteric fracture. She has insulin-dependent diabetes mellitus as well as previous renal transplant. The risks, benefits, and alternatives to left bipolar hemiarthroplasty were discussed with her and she agreed to proceed.

PROCEDURE: The patient was brought to the operating room, placed under spinal anesthesia, and received preoperative antibiotics. Her left hip was prepped and draped in the usual sterile manner. Incision was made over the proximal femur and taken down to subcutaneous tissue to fascia. The fascia was split in line with the skin incision. An anterior lateral Harding approach was utilized. The capsule was T'd. The proximal femur was exposed. Again there was a displaced femoral neck fracture. I used a template to initially make my neck cut. I subsequently removed the head with corkscrew. This was sized to size 41, used a trial 41 within the acetabular component and this fit well. I left the labrum but did take out the ligamentum teres. The hip was thoroughly irrigated. I then subsequently turned my attention to the proximal femur. A starting reamer was utilized. I utilized a lateralizer. I subsequently reamed to size 5. Overall I had very good fit. I actually broached one size over my axial reaming. The broach fit well. I subsequently placed a +5 trial head, a 41 trial acetabular component, and reduced the hip, and overall the leg length looked well. There was perhaps just a slight increased length as compared with the right but overall leg length stability. I was happy with the overall position and alignment. I subsequently dislocated the hip, removed the component. The canal was thoroughly irrigated; Raytecs were placed in the canal. I subsequently cemented in the real stem with a +5 neck with a 41-mm bipolar component. The real trials were utilized. I did also utilize a cement restrictor and a centralizer. The hip was thoroughly irrigated. The abductors were closed to the greater trochanter using #5 Ethibond. The fascia was closed with 0 Vicryl, skin was closed with subcutaneous Z–0 Vicryl, 3–0 Monocryl for skin as well as staples. She was placed in a sterile dressing, awakened, and taken to recovery uneventfully. She tolerated the above operative procedure with no known complications. Estimated blood loss was 200 cc.

PLAN: We will allow her to weight-bear as tolerated and get her mobilized tomorrow. We will keep her for closer monitoring overnight in the intensive care unit and likely hopefully transfer to the orthopedic floor tomorrow.

PROGRESS NOTE

LOCATION: Inpatient, Hospital

PATIENT: Dina Olson

ATTENDING PHYSICIAN: Laddie N. Noss, MD

The patient is seen today. Her postoperative pain is being controlled with morphine. The hip seems to be doing well. She has been transferred from the ICU to the floor. She has essentially stabilized. Again, the belief is that she is likely having some type of seizure activity.

PHYSICAL EXAMINATION: Her vitals overall are fairly well stabilized. Her postoperative dressings are in place. She did have a significantly elevated INR, so the dressings have been kept in place to minimize the risk for bleeding. She was sleeping when I saw her, so I did not wake her. Her toes are pink and warm. Calves are soft.

IMPRESSION: Status post left hip bipolar hemiarthroplasty.

PLAN: From my standpoint, she can mobilize and weight bear as tolerated on the left side. We will change her dressings and place TED hose on the left. We will continue to follow her INR and hemoglobin. Of note, she has been made code status II.

DISCHARGE SUMMARY

LOCATION: Inpatient, Hospital

PATIENT: Dina Olson

ATTENDING PHYSICIAN: Laddie N. Noss, MD

This patient was admitted after an accidental fall at home. She had a displaced left femoral neck fracture and underwent left bipolar hip replacement. Her postoperative course was characterized by a decreased mental status, which I feel was ultimately due to breakthrough seizures, which were finally diagnosed by EEG. She subsequently has improved on Dilantin control. Her brain MRI did not show any abnormality. Since therapy, her mental status has pretty much approached normal. She is eating better. We had problems with her consistently eating but that seems to be resolving. Her diabetes is under excellent control. We are actually increasing slightly her Glargine and NovoLog regimen. The Glargine is up to 5 and NovoLog 5, if she eats a full meal. If she does not eat a meal, the NovoLog will not be given. If she eats a partial meal, the nurse has the option of giving a little bit less insulin, such as 3 units. That will be titrated as needed. The Dilantin level was being obtained and neurology will adjust that. Her dialysis regimen is going well. She is on 4-hour runs three times a week—Monday, Wednesday, and Friday. Her Coumadin and anticoagulation is progressing nicely as well.

The long-term question post rehab will be whether she is capable of independent living and self-care. That is one of the main concerns at this time. We will address that with the rehab personnel as well as the patient and her family.

FINAL DIAGNOSES
1. Displaced femoral neck fracture of hip, status post bipolar hip replacement.
2. Seizure disorder.
3. End-stage renal disease secondary to diabetic nephropathy.
4. Chronic maintenance hemodialysis.
5. Type I diabetes.
6. Diabetic nephropathy.
7. Diabetes gastroparesis.
8. Diabetic retinopathy.
9. Anemia of chronic disease.

Total time spent preparing summary, discussing management with consultants, and counseling patient was 50 minutes, from 2:00 PM to 2:50 PM.

CPT Code(s): _____

ICD-9-CM Code(s): _____

ICD-10-CM Code(s): _____

Abstracting Questions

1. What is the primary reason for this admission? _____

2. What medical conditions existed at the time of admission that affected management of the patient?

   _____

3. What other medical condition presented during the patient's stay? _____

4. Are E codes reported to describe how and where injury occurred? _____

5. Is time a factor in coding the discharge? _____

Case 115: Breast Cancer

There are three reports that are to be considered when coding this hospital stay.

HISTORY AND PHYSICAL EXAM

LOCATION: Inpatient, Hospital

PATIENT: Constance Noyes

ATTENDING PHYSICIAN: Alma Naraquist, MD

This is a 76-year-old female with metastatic breast cancer.

The patient was discharged on the 19th following stent placement on the 18th. The patient's CT on the 22nd still showed some hydronephrosis.

In any event, the patient has continued to become progressively uremic, now her creatinine is over 8. She has advanced uremic symptoms, including decreased mental capacity.

PAST MEDICAL HISTORY: Notable for breast cancer, about 14 years ago left breast was removed. I understand she had tumors twice in that breast.

She has had hypertension and back pain with tumors metastatic to the spine. Radiation to this area has caused the retroperitoneal fibrosis and ureteric obstruction. She has a history of hypothyroidism, gastroesophageal reflux disease, and anemia.

SURGICAL HISTORY
1. Lumbar depression.
2. Open cholecystectomy.
3. Right cataract extraction.
4. Multiple lucencies.
5. Right total hip arthroplasty.
6. Vein stripping.
7. Left mastectomy.

SOCIAL HISTORY: She is widowed and lives independently.

FAMILY HISTORY: Father died possibly from prostate cancer and pulmonary embolism.

MEDICATIONS: have been
1. Dexamethasone 0.75 mg b.i.d.
2. Oxycodone 10 mg every 4 to 6 hours as required; that is, the CR OxyContin.
3. Protonix 40 mg daily.
4. Taxotere last in November.
5. She has been on Zoloft 50 mg daily.
6. She has been on Zometa, which is a biphosphonate 40 mg, and this probably has not been helpful in the setting of renal failure.

ALLERGIES: Contrast, codeine, penicillin, and morphine.

SYSTEMS REVIEW: The patient has been confused. She had a fall. Balance has been poor. She has eaten practically nothing. Weight is down. She had an emesis this morning. Appetite has dwindled to pretty much nothing. Interestingly, at this time, she does not have any back or bone pain.

EXAMINATION: Notable for a patient who is pleasantly confused. She knows her name and where she lives. She knows who the president is, but does not know who the mayor is. She is reasonably oriented to place and person. She knows this is the hospital, but she has a peculiar type of speech and way of expressing herself, which is certainly strange and not normal, so the patient certainly is not right. Dr. Boe has already done a CT, and there is no metastatic lesion in the head. The patient's blood pressure is 155/80 with a temperature of 37.8°C. Pulse rate was 80 and the patient does not have edema. Left breast is absent. The heart sounds are unremarkable. No carotid bruits. Respiratory system: Trachea central. The breath sounds are reasonably clear. Mouth is dry. Right breast is normal. The abdomen is quite abnormal. There is hardness over the abdomen especially centrally up into the right. There are nodular masses easily palpable, and I am pretty sure I am feeling a knotted mass of mesentery. She does have bowel sounds.

The patient moves all four limbs.

I did have an ultrasound done. She still has some hydronephrosis of both kidneys, mild to moderate, but I think this is just because she has been hydronephrotic so long it does not go down to normal.

The patient is in advanced renal failure. BUN is 65 and creatinine is 8.3. Total CO_2 is down to 14.3, so she has significant metabolic acidosis. Sodium is diluted 129 and potassium is 5.1. CPK is normal. White count is normal. Hemoglobin is 10.

This patient is 76. She has a widely metastatic breast cancer. Abdomen has a very ominous feel to it.

Her CT has been without contrast, and they have noticed abnormal stranding in the mesentery and I think they have been looking at tumor. Her clinical examination is much more impressive than the CT.

I have explained the situation to her daughter that we are in a code II designation but really I think we are close to III.

I have a hard time placing burden of care in this situation of going to dialysis in her situation. It is unlikely the renal situation will turn around. I think probably the less we do for this patient the better. We need to concentrate on keeping her comfortable and I think she will likely succumb shortly whatever we do and I think it better that she succumb without excessive interference of medical management.

At this time, then, we have a patient with metastatic breast cancer to the spine and into the abdomen by clinical examination. She now has established renal failure with significant uremia. This is both by lab and symptomatically. The patient is certainly in a feeble, weakened state. The patient will be admitted to the hospitalist service as above. I have spent an hour evaluating this patient this evening.

OPERATIVE REPORT

LOCATION: Inpatient, Hospital

PATIENT: Constance Noyes

ATTENDING PHYSICIAN: Alma Naraquist, MD

SURGEON: Ira Avila, MD

PREOPERATIVE DIAGNOSIS: Acute renal failure, bilateral ureteropelvic junction obstruction.

POSTOPERATIVE DIAGNOSIS: Acute renal failure, bilateral ureteropelvic junction obstruction.

PROCEDURE PERFORMED: Cystoscopy, bilateral ureteral stent change.

DESCRIPTION OF PROCEDURE: The patient was given IV sedation and prepped and draped position. Urethra anesthetized with 2% Xylocaine jelly. A 21 French cystoscope passed into the bladder under direct vision. Stents were grasped and removed to urethral meatus. Guidewires were advanced up the stent and the stents exchanged for 8 French 26 cm stents bilaterally. Fluoroscopic control was used. Conray was injected in a retrograde fashion through an open-ended ureteral catheter that was placed over the guidewires to identify collecting systems. There was no obvious abnormality. There was persistence of the upper ureteral stenosis secondary to retroperitoneal lymphadenopathy. The patient tolerated the procedure well, and a Foley catheter was not replaced. She was transferred to the recovery room in good condition.

DISCHARGE SUMMARY

LOCATION: Inpatient, Hospital

PATIENT: Constance Noyes

ATTENDING PHYSICIAN: Alma Naraquist, MD

FINAL DIAGNOSES
 1. Metastatic breast carcinoma.
 2. Acute renal failure.
 3. Altered mental status.
 4. Nausea and vomiting.
 5. Hypocalcemia, hypomagnesemia, hypophosphatemia.
 6. Anorexia.
 7. Malnutrition.
 8. Hypoalbuminemia.
 9. Pain syndrome.
10. Deconditioning and debilitation.
11. Subcutaneous nodule, possible metastatic breast cancer.
12. Anemia secondary to chronic disease.

CONDITION ON DISCHARGE: Improved.

DISPOSITION: The patient will be discharged. Follow-up blood counts, chemistry including CMP, magnesium, phosphorus, and ionized calcium. Additional IV hydration may be required. She may need to be brought to the office on that day.

HOSPITAL COURSE: The patient is known to have breast carcinoma for about 10 years. She had been on salvage treatment with Taxotere. That had been discontinued in November, when it was believed the disease was stable. The disease had been found to be metastatic to the spine. She had radiation, and it was believed she was developing retroperitoneal fibrosis and ureteric obstruction. She also has a history of hypothyroidism, GERD, and anemia. On admission she was found to be confused. This was attributed to decreased excretion of her narcotic medications. After improvement of renal function, her confusion resolved. The chemotherapy was relatively well tolerated. She had some problems with constipation. Those have resolved. The renal failure was managed with active hydration and by the time of discharge, kidney function was normal. She required multiple electrolyte replacement. Nutrition still remains a problem. She will continue further dietary supplements as needed. There had been also initial body deconditioning. Physical therapy and occupational therapy had started working with her.

CPT Code(s): _____

ICD-9-CM Code(s): _____

ICD-10-CM Code(s): _____

Abstracting Questions

1. What is the principal admitting diagnosis? _____

2. For what condition was the procedure performed? _____

3. Are the patient's various metabolic and other conditions reported? _____

4. How is the cystoscopy with stent placement reported? _____

5. Are the neoplastic diagnoses reported? _____

Case 116: Groin Pain

There are 10 reports that are to be considered when coding this hospital stay.

HISTORY AND PHYSICAL EXAM (INTERNAL MEDICINE)

LOCATION: Inpatient, Hospital

PATIENT: Emma Detlaff

ATTENDING PHYSICIAN: Alma Naraquist, MD

This patient is 62 years old. She has significant vascular disease and renal disease. She is on peritoneal dialysis. She has had numerous stents placed in her heart and also stents in her lower extremities. She has had a bypass surgery for circulation in her lower legs.

Her main complaint today is that she has pain in her right groin area, which makes it impossible for her to walk. Because of the pain, she had significant difficulties getting dressed this morning. She performed one run of peritoneal dialysis today. She usually does this four times per day.

This pain is sharp and has been gradually progressive over the past two weeks. The severity is 7 out of 10, which was much worse today and prompted her to come in.

PAST MEDICAL HISTORY: As mentioned above, she has the significant vascular disease. She also has diabetes, hyperlipidemia, and hypertension. She has a decreased ejection fraction. She has had cataracts removed, carpal tunnel surgery, and a hysterectomy. She has also had three brain aneurysm surgeries.

ALLERGIES: Penicillin and Ticlid.

CURRENT MEDICATIONS
1. Coumadin 5 mg/day.
2. Insulin: Humalog 40 units in the morning, 20 units at 1 PM, and 25 units at 4:30 PM.
3. Potassium 10 mEq twice a day.
4. Lanoxin 0.125 mg/day.
5. Nifedipine 30 mg daily.
6. Pravachol 20 at h.s.
7. Renagel 800 mg one t.i.d.

FAMILY HISTORY: She has a son who is diabetic and had a kidney transplant. Father passed away from Alzheimer disease. Mother had heart disease.

SOCIAL HISTORY: She continues to smoke.

REVIEW OF SYSTEMS: She denies chest pain or worsening shortness of breath. She has been having regular bowel movements. She denies loss of appetite. She has not eaten much today because of her inability to ambulate. She reports that she does make urine. Her peritoneal dialysis has been going well of late.

PHYSICAL EXAMINATION: This lady is sitting on an exam gurney and looks to be in no distress. She claims to have severe pain in her groin but looks rather calm and collected. Blood pressure 125/58, afebrile, pulse in the 60s and regular, 99% saturation on room air. I do not appreciate any JVD in the neck. No carotid bruits. LUNGS: Fair air exchange without wheezes or crackles. HEART: Irregularly irregular. ABDOMEN: Mildly distended. There are active bowel sounds. Peritoneal dialysis tubing is clean and taped to the abdomen. No evidence of ecchymosis or swelling in the right groin. She has pain when I palpate that area. I can feel a femoral pulse. I do not appreciate any abnormal mass. She is also tender over the greater trochanter of the hip. Flexing the hip is painful for her but can be done. She has warm feet with palpable dorsalis pedis pulse in both feet. No significant edema.

Her white count is 16,000, hemoglobin 11.9, platelet count 263,000. She has 81% neutrophils, 13% lymphocytes. BUN 24, creatinine 3.1, sodium 132, potassium 3.2, blood sugar 102, protime 15 seconds with an INR of 1.8.

X-rays of the hip reveal demineralized bone but no obvious fracture.

IMPRESSION: A 62-year-old lady with:
1. Severe right groin pain.
2. Inability to ambulate secondary to #1.
3. Chronic renal failure.
4. Peritoneal dialysis.
5. Severe vascular disease.
6. Leukocytosis.
7. Hyponatremia.
8. Hypokalemia.

PLAN: I am puzzled as to the etiology of this discomfort. She probably needs a bone scan. I do not think we can do an MRI because of her previous vascular surgeries and staples. We can treat the pain with morphine. I talked a bit about code status. She was fairly noncommittal and said that she would put that in her family's hands. Right now, we would have to keep her code I based on that conversation.

RADIOLOGY REPORT (RADIOLOGIST)

LOCATION: Inpatient, Hospital

PATIENT: Emma Detlaff

ATTENDING PHYSICIAN: Alma Naraquist, MD

RADIOLOGIST: Morton Monson, MD

EXAMINATION OF: Pelvis/hip.

CLINICAL SYMPTOMS: Right groin pain.

PELVIS AND RIGHT HIP, TWO VIEWS: Within all of the osseous structures. The radiopaque Tenckhoff catheters. There is ASVD, and left iliac stent is noted.

On evaluation of the bony structures, the obturator rings I believe are basically intact. There is demineralization within the osseous structures. The iliac wings and right hip as visualized appear to be intact. I do not see specific fracture displacement.

CONCLUSION
1. Demineralization within all of the osseous structures making assessment difficult. I do not believe that there is specific fracture displacement involving portions of the pelvis or right hip that is evaluated.
2. If the patient has persistent clinical symptomatology, follow-up evaluation or other imaging studies such as MR or bone scan may be considered.

3. Incidental finding of heavy aortoiliac and lower extremity ASVD. An iliac stent is noted on the left.
4. Radiopaque Tenckhoff catheter superimposes the pelvis.

DIALYSIS PROGRESS NOTE (NEPHROLOGIST)

LOCATION: Inpatient, Hospital

PATIENT: Emma Detlaff

ATTENDING PHYSICIAN: Gordon Jayco, MD

The patient was seen during peritoneal dialysis. We are using 1.5% alternating with 2.5%. Her dialysate looked clear when we did the last exchange. We are using 2-liter fill volumes, 4 exchanges a day.

She was admitted earlier with severe right hip pain and she was not able to move or walk. She did have that 2 weeks ago. I advised her to have an x-ray and have an evaluation, but she declined at that time. I saw her today, and she has had tenderness in the inguinal area. Her tenderness is probably coming from her right hip. Her x-ray was negative, however, for any obvious fractures.

The patient looks very cachectic and has lost at least 7 to 9 pounds in the past 2 weeks. This could be related to the amount of pain she is having and her not eating, but I would be worried about malignancy in this situation. It is worth mentioning that she has chronic leukocytosis.

She is a dialysis patient with CRF and is expected to have secondary hyperparathyroidism. She could have a subtle fracture or metastatic disease. She is not a candidate for MRI because of her previous brain surgery and aneurysm clipping. We will proceed with a bone scan on Monday. I discussed this with the internal medicine physician and he was in agreement. I will continue to follow her from the dialysis standpoint.

Thank you for allowing me to participate in the care of this patient.

PROGRESS NOTE (INTERNAL MEDICINE)

LOCATION: Inpatient, Hospital

PATIENT: Emma Detlaff

ATTENDING PHYSICIAN: Alma Naraquist, MD

SUBJECTIVE: Continues to have a great deal of right groin pain. Pain was quite unbearable this morning, trying to get to the bathroom. She has not been running a fever. She did have some nausea and vomiting from the morphine. No diarrhea. No other areas of bony pain.

OBJECTIVE: Temperature 35.8, blood pressure 106/42, pulse 78, respirations 18, O_2 saturations 98%. Generally alert and oriented, appears uncomfortable. Chest clear; no rales, rhonchi, or wheezing. Heart fairly regular and rhythm. Abdomen is protuberant.

ASSESSMENT
1. Severe persistent right groin pain.
2. Diabetes mellitus.
3. Coronary artery disease.
4. Peripheral vascular disease.

PLAN: She has a bone scan scheduled for today. Depending on how that looks, will make decision regarding CT scan.

RADIOLOGY REPORT (RADIOLOGIST)

LOCATION: Inpatient, Hospital

PATIENT: Emma Detlaff

ATTENDING PHYSICIAN: Alma Naraquist, MD

RADIOLOGIST: Morton Monson, MD

EXAMINATION OF: Radionuclide bone scan, whole-body scan.

CLINICAL SYMPTOMS: Right groin pain.

RADIONUCLIDE BONE SCAN: Dose: The patient received 27 millicuries technetium-99m HDP intravenously.

FINDINGS: This examination is compared with a prior radionuclide bone scan. Whole-body bone scan was performed today. There is some apparent increased activity seen to involve the right hemipelvis in the area of the right superior and inferior pubic rami. There is, however, urinary bladder activity immediately adjacent to this, which makes the evaluation somewhat difficult. This does appear to be different from the prior study, and findings are highly suspicious for insufficiency fractures involving the right inferior and superior pubic rami. There is new focal intense activity involving the lateral femoral condyle of the right femur. Posttraumatic causes are considered to be most likely; however, other causes are not excluded. Close clinical correlation is suggested. Asymmetric renal activity is noted, which is similar to the prior study. Abnormal activity involves both shoulders, in a pattern most consistent with arthritic change.

IMPRESSION
1. Increased activity noted within the right hemipelvis, as discussed above. Findings are believed to be most compatible with insufficiency fracture. Correlate that finding clinically. Visualization is limited by the presence of adjacent urinary bladder activity.
2. New focus of intense abnormal activity involving the distal right femur. That is believed to most likely be posttraumatic in nature. Again, close clinical correlation is suggested.
3. Scattered arthritic changes, as described.

DIALYSIS PROGRESS NOTE (NEPHROLOGIST)

LOCATION: Inpatient, Hospital

PATIENT: Emma Detlaff

ATTENDING PHYSICIAN: Alma Naraquist, MD

NEPHROLOGIST: Gordon Jayco, MD

The patient was seen on peritoneal dialysis. We are using 1.5 alternating with 2.5%. She had no ultrafiltration this morning. She was subsequently seen 1.5 hours into the dialysis today. She continues to have right hip pain, and she is going to have a bone scan done today. She appears euvolemic on physical examination, and we will continue with the current dialysis prescription.

She has not required any hydromorphone. She received Compazine for nausea.

The patient agrees with the plan.

PROGRESS NOTE (INTERNAL MEDICINE)

LOCATION: Inpatient, Hospital

PATIENT: Emma Detlaff

ATTENDING PHYSICIAN: Alma Naraquist, MD

SUBJECTIVE: She is still having a great deal of pain with movement.

She just learned recently that her husband has neck cancer and decisions are pending regarding treatment.

OBJECTIVE: TEMPERATURE: 36.4. BLOOD PRESSURE: 112/40. PULSE: 87. RESPIRATIONS: 18. O$_2$ SATS: 96%. Generally, appears fairly comfortable. CHEST: Clear to auscultation. No rales, rhonchi, or wheezing. HEART: Regular rate and rhythm. Bone scan shows fracture of her pelvis in the right superior and inferior pubis ramus.

ASSESSMENT
1. Atraumatic pelvic fracture.
2. Severe persistent right groin pain secondary to #1.
3. Diabetes mellitus.
4. Coronary artery disease.
5. Peripheral vascular disease.
6. End-stage renal disease.

PLAN: Consultation with orthopedic surgeon. She will need to be limited in her mobility for probably 6 to 8 weeks, using either a walker or crutches. We are tentatively planning on transfer to a nursing home within the next couple of days. We will have PT and OT work with her. We will need to educate the nursing home staff about her peritoneal dialysis. We will see about getting some oral pain meds for her. We will check to see when her most recent DEXA scan was to evaluate the osteoporosis concern.

DIALYSIS PROGRESS NOTE (NEPHROLOGIST)

LOCATION: Inpatient, Hospital

PATIENT: Emma Detlaff

ATTENDING PHYSICIAN: Alma Naraquist, MD

NEPHROLOGIST: Gordon Jayco, MD

The patient was seen on CAPD. We are using 1.5% alternating with 2.5%, 2-liter fill volumes with insulin. Yesterday she had 450 out. Her exchange today is not done yet.

The patient had a pelvic fracture on the right side on the bone scan. She needs probably bedrest for a while. We will discuss whether he wants to proceed with a CT. I talked to Social Services to discuss options for discharge including nursing home placement. I also addressed that issue with the patient. Meanwhile will continue current dialysis prescription, and from the nutrition standpoint we will give her high-protein Boost t.i.d.

PROGRESS NOTE (INTERNAL MEDICINE)

LOCATION: Inpatient, Hospital

PATIENT: Emma Detlaff

ATTENDING PHYSICIAN: Alma Naraquist, MD

SUBJECTIVE: Continues to have right hip pain, but codeine, which we ordered, does seem to work well for her. She continues to have pain in both shin areas.

OBJECTIVE: Temp 36.2, pulse 90, respirations 20, blood pressure 122/46. Chest: Normal respiratory effort, clear to auscultation. Heart: Regular rate and rhythm.

Sugars yesterday were 318, 294, 245, and 329; today 264.

ASSESSMENT
1. Atraumatic right pelvic fracture.
2. Right groin pain secondary to #1.
3. Diabetes mellitus.
4. Coronary artery disease.
5. Peripheral vascular disease.
6. End-stage renal disease.

PLAN: Nursing home has accepted her and tentatively a bed will be available this coming Friday, the 7th of May. Will try some cold packs to her shin areas. Will continue with PT and OT.

DISCHARGE SUMMARY (INTERNAL MEDICINE)

LOCATION: Inpatient, Hospital

PATIENT: Emma Detlaff

ATTENDING PHYSICIAN: Alma Naraquist, MD

REASON FOR ADMISSION: Severe right groin pain.

HISTORY OF PRESENT ILLNESS/PHYSICAL EXAMINATION: See admission history and physical (H&P) examination.

LABORATORY DATA: Metabolic panel showed a sodium of 132, chloride 93, potassium 3.2, BUN 24, and creatinine 3.1. Comprehensive panel shows a sodium 133, chloride 95, potassium 3.2, BUN 24, creatinine 3.1, alkaline phosphatase 190. Sugars on the day of admission 90 and 203, and on the day of discharge 162 and 181. CPK was normal. CBC showed hemoglobin 11.9 and white count of 16.6.

X-RAY: X-ray of the right hip and pelvis showed some demineralization; otherwise, no specific fracture. Bone scan showed increased activity in the right hemipelvis consistent with fracture in the superior and inferior pubic ramus.

HOSPITAL COURSE AND TREATMENT: The patient was admitted with the right groin pain; severe, persistent. She was continued on her medications, placed on bed rest, and bone scan was ordered. Nephrologist saw her and managed her fluids. The return of the bone scan showing a fracture, PT/OT was consulted. She was given codeine for pain and consultation with the orthopedic surgeon. He recommended conservative management with use of a walker. Because of her current living situation, arrangements were made for her to be transferred to the nursing home and recuperate there.

TRANSFER MEDICATIONS
1. Calcitrol 0.25 daily.
2. Digoxin 0.125 daily.
3. Epogen 1000 units every Thursday.
4. Nifedipine XL 30 mg daily.
5. Potassium 10 mEq t.i.d.
6. Pravachol 20 mg at bedtime.
7. Renagel 800 t.i.d.
8. Coumadin 3 mg daily.
9. Reglan 10 mg q.i.d.
10. Acetaminophen 500 mg daily.
11. Calcium carbonate p.r.n.
12. Codeine 30 to 60 mg p.o. q.i.d. p.r.n.
13. Insulin 40 units in the morning, 20 at 1:00 PM, and 25 at 4:30 PM.

DISCHARGE RECOMMENDATION AND FOLLOW-UP: She is to continue on her diabetic diet, checking sugars at the nursing home. She is to gradually increase her weight-bearing, depending on the pain level in her pelvis. OT and PT will see her.

FINAL DIAGNOSES
1. Atraumatic right pelvic fracture.
2. Diabetes mellitus type 1.
3. Coronary artery disease.
4. Peripheral vascular disease.
5. End-stage renal disease.
6. Hyperlipidemia.
7. Hypertension.
8. Chronic tobacco abuse.
9. Chronic anticoagulation.
10. Chronic leukocytosis.

CPT Code(s): _____

ICD-9-CM Code(s): _____

ICD-10-CM Code(s): _____

Abstracting Questions

1. Is the admitting presenting problem reported as the principal diagnosis? _____

2. What is the principal diagnosis for this admission? _____

3. Was there surgical management of the fracture? _____

4. Are the patient's chronic conditions reported for this stay? _____

5. Are the various metabolic issues in the H&P reported? _____

6. Does the patient have anticoagulant management to be reported? _____

7. What type of procedure was done during the patient's stay? _____

Appendix
Coding Answers to Patient Cases

CHAPTER 1: INTEGUMENTARY

Case 1
Facility: 14060 (Tissue Transfer, Adjacent, Skin);
173.3 (Neoplasm, skin, nose [external], Malignant, Primary)

ICD-10-CM: C44.31 (Neoplasm, skin, nose [external], Malignant, Primary)

Case 2
Facility: 13101 (Repair, Skin, Wound, Complex, Trunk, 2.6 cm-7.5 cm) and **+13102** (each additional 5 cm or less); **707.8** (Ulcer, hip)

ICD-10-CM: L98.499 (Ulcer, skin, specified site)

Case 3
Facility: 11043 (Debridement, Muscle); **707.09** (Ulcer, decubitus, other site), **707.24** (Ulcer, pressure, stage IV)

ICD-10-CM: L89.894 (Ulcer, pressure [area], specified site)

Case 4
Facility: 97605 (Wound, Negative Pressure Therapy); **V58.31** (Attention [to], surgical dressings)

ICD-10-CM: Z48.01 (Attention to, surgical dressings)

Case 5
Facility: 15120 (Skin Graft and Flap, Split Graft); **707.15** (Ulcer, lower extremity, foot), **707.13** (Ulcer, lower extremity, ankle)

ICD-10-CM: L97.511 (Ulcer, lower limb, foot, right, with, skin breakdown only), **L97.311** (Ulcer, lower limb, ankle, right, with, skin breakdown only)

Case 6
Facility: 97605 (Negative Pressure Wound Therapy), **11043** (Debridement, Muscle), **11042-59** (Debridement, Subcutaneous Tissue); **707.15** (Ulcer, lower extremity, foot), **707.14** (Ulcer, lower

extremity, heel), **V58.31** (Attention to surgical dressings)

ICD-10-CM: L97.512 (Ulcer, lower limb, foot, with, exposed fat layer), **L97.421** (Ulcer, lower limb, heel, with, skin breakdown only), **Z48.01** (Admission [for], change of surgical dressings)

Case 7
Facility: 11402 (Excision, Skin, Lesion, Benign); **216.5** (Neoplasm, skin, chest [wall], Benign)

ICD-10-CM: D22.5 (Nevus, skin, chest wall)

Case 8
Facility: 10061 (Drainage, Skin; Incision and Drainage of Abscess, Multiple); **682.3** (Abscess, arm), **686.9** (Pustule)

ICD-10-CM: L02.414 (Abscess, upper limb), **L08.9** (Pustule)

CHAPTER 2: GASTROINTESTINAL

Case 9
Facility: 45330 (Sigmoidoscopy, Exploration); **009.0** (Colitis, infectious), **780.60** (Fever)

ICD-10-CM: A09 (Enteritis, infectious NOS), **R50.9** (Fever)

Case 10
Facility: 45380 (Colonoscopy, Biopsy); **787.91** (Diarrhea), **789.00** (Cramp[s], abdominal), **787.01** (Nausea, with vomiting)

ICD-10-CM: R19.7 (Diarrhea), **R10.84** (Pain, abdominal, generalized), **R11.2** (Nausea, with vomiting)

Case 11
Facility: 43239 (Endoscopy, Gastrointestinal, Upper, Biopsy); **535.51** (Gastritis, with hemorrhage)

ICD-10-CM: K29.71 (Gastritis, with bleeding)

Case 12
Facility: 45330 (Sigmoidoscopy, Exploration); **792.1** (Findings, abnormal, without diagnosis, stool, occult blood), **285.9** (Anemia), **562.10** (Diverticula, sigmoid)

ICD-10-CM: R19.5 (Occult, blood in feces [stools]), **D64.9** (Anemia), **K57.30** (Diverticulosis, large intestine)

Case 13
Facility: 44388 (Colonoscopy, via Stoma); **578.9** (Hemorrhage, gastrointestinal [tract])

ICD-10-CM: K92.2 (Hemorrhage, gastrointestinal (tract))

Case 14
Facility: 45384 (Colonoscopy, Removal Polyp); **153.3** (Neoplasm, intestine, large, colon, sigmoid [flexure], Malignant, Primary), **211.3** (Neoplasm, intestine, large, colon, ascending, Benign)

ICD-10-CM: C18.7 (Neoplasm, intestine, large, colon, sigmoid (flexure), Malignant Primary), **D12.2** (Neoplasm, intestine, large, colon, ascending, Benign), **D12.3** (Neoplasm, intestine, large, colon, transverse, Malignant Primary)

Case 15
Facility: 45385 (Colonoscopy, Removal, Polyp), **45384-59** (Colonoscopy, Removal, Polyp); **211.3** (Neoplasm, intestine, large, colon, sigmoid, Benign), **562.10** (Diverticula, sigmoid)

ICD-10-CM: D12.5 (Neoplasm, intestine, large, colon, sigmoid, Benign), **K57.30** (Diverticulosis, large intestine)

Case 16
Facility: 43235 (Endoscopy, Gastrointestinal, Upper, Exploration); **793.4** (Findings, abnormal, without diagnosis, radiologic, gastrointestinal tract), **787.20** (Dysphagia)

ICD-10-CM: R93.3 (Findings, abnormal, without diagnosis, radiologic, gastrointestinal tract), **R13.10** (Dysphagia)

Case 17
Facility: 45380 (Colonoscopy, Biopsy); **792.1** (Findings, abnormal, without diagnosis, stool, occult blood), **455.0** (Hemorrhoids, internal)

ICD-10-CM: R19.5 (Occult, blood in feces [stools]), **I84.21** (Hemorrhoids, internal)

CHAPTER 3: NEPHROLOGY

Case 18
Facility: 36514 (Apheresis, Therapeutic); **358.00** (Myasthenia)

ICD-10-CM: G70.00 (Myasthenia, gravis)

Case 19
Facility: 50200-RT (Biopsy, Kidney), **76942** (Ultrasound, Guidance, Needle Biopsy); **580.4** (Nephritis, necrotizing, acute), **V42.0** (Status (post), transplant, kidney)

ICD-10-CM: N00.8 (Glomerulonephritis, necrotic, necrotizing, NEC), **Z94.0** (Transplant, kidney)

Case 20
Facility: 36514 (Apheresis, Therapeutic); **358.00** (Myasthenia)

ICD-10-CM: G70.00 (Myasthenia, gravis)

Case 21
Facility: 50200-RT (Biopsy, Kidney), **76942** (Ultrasound, Guidance, Needle Biopsy); **583.1** (Glomerulonephritis, membranous)

ICD-10-CM: N05.2 (Glomerulonephritis, membranous NEC)

Case 22
Facility: 36558 (Insertion, Catheter, Venous); **584.9** (Failure, renal, acute)

ICD-10-CM: N17.9 (Failure, renal, acute)

CHAPTER 4: NEUROLOGY/NEUROSURGERY

Case 23
Facility: 62270 (Spinal Tap, Lumbar); **784.0** (Headache)

ICD-10-CM: R51 (Headache)

Case 24
Facility: 95816 (Electroencephalography [EEG], Standard); **794.02** (Findings, abnormal, without diagnosis, electroencephalogram [EEG]), **780.39** (Seizure)

ICD-10-CM: R94.01 (Abnormal, electroencephalogram [EEG]), **R56.9** (Seizure)

Case 25
Facility: 64721-LT (Release, Carpal Tunnel); **354.0** (Syndrome, carpal tunnel)

ICD-10-CM: G56.02 (Syndrome, carpal tunnel)

Case 26
Facility: 63030-LT (Hemilaminectomy); **722.10** (Displacement, intervertebral disc, lumbar, lumbosacral)

ICD-10-CM: M51.27 (Displacement, intervertebral disc, lumbosacral region)

Case 27
Facility: 61020 (Ventricular, Puncture); **191.6** (Neoplasm, cerebellum NOS, Malignant, Primary), **331.4** (Hydrocephalus [obstructive])

ICD-10-CM: C71.6 (Neoplasm, cerebellum NOS, Malignant Primary), **G91.4** (Hydrocephalus, in neoplastic disease NEC)

Case 28
Facility: 95816 (Electroencephalography [EEG]); **294.8** (Dementia)

ICD-10-CM: F03 (Dementia)

Case 29
Facility: 62350 (Insertion, Catheter, Spinal Cord), **62362** (Insertion, Infusion Pump, Spinal Cord); **733.00** (Osteoporosis), **724.02** (Stenosis, spinal, lumbar, lumbosacral), **722.52** (Degeneration, intervertebral disc, lumbar, lumbosacral)

ICD-10-CM: M81.0 (Osteoporosis, specific type NEC), **M48.06** (Stenosis, spinal, lumbar region), **M51.36** (Degeneration, intervertebral disc, lumbar region)

CHAPTER 5: OBSTETRIC AND GYNECOLOGIC SURGERY AND OPHTHALMOLOGY

Case 30
Facility: 58558 (Hysteroscopy, Surgical, with Biopsy); **621.0** (Polyp, endometrium)

ICD-10-CM: N84.0 (Polyp, endometrium)

Case 31
Facility: 59000 (Amniocentesis), **76946** (Ultrasound, Guidance, Amniocentesis); **V28.2** (Screening, antenatal, of mother, based on amniocentesis), **648.03** (Pregnancy, complicated, diabetes, antepartum), **250.40** (Diabetes, nephropathy), **583.81** (Nephropathy, diabetic), **V58.67** (Long-term [current] drug use, insulin)

ICD-10-CM: Z36 (Screening, antenatal, of mother), **O24.113** (Pregnancy, complicated by, diabetes, pre-existing, type 2), **E11.21** (Diabetes, type 2, with nephropathy), **Z79.4** (Long-term [current] drug therapy [use of] insulin)

Case 32
Facility: 68720 (Dacryocystorhinostomy); **375.42** (Dacryocystitis, chronic)

ICD-10-CM: H04.412 (Dacryocystitis, chronic)

Case 33
Facility: 67923-E1, 67923-E3 (Repair, Eyelid, Entropion, Excision Tarsal Wedge); **374.00** (Entropion, eyelid)

ICD-10-CM: H02.001 (Entropion [eyelid], right, upper), **H02.004** (Entropion [eyelid], left, upper)

Case 34
Facility: 68110 (Excision, Lesion, Conjunctiva); **372.00** (Caruncle [inflamed], conjunctiva)

ICD-10-CM: H10.31 (Conjunctivitis, acute)

CHAPTER 6: ORTHOPEDIC

Case 35
Facility: 29888-RT (Arthroscopy, Surgical, Knee); **717.83** (Derangement, cruciate ligament [knee], anterior)

ICD-10-CM: M23.611 (Derangement, knee, ligament, anterior cruciate)

Case 36
Facility: 29880-RT (Arthroscopy, Surgical, Knee), **29877-RT** (Arthroscopy, Surgical, Knee); **836.0** (Tear, meniscus, medial, posterior horn), **836.1** (Tear, meniscus, lateral), **715.96** (Osteoarthrosis, lower leg)

ICD-10-CM: S83.241A (Tear, meniscus [knee], medial, specified type NEC), **S83.281A** (Tear, meniscus [knee], lateral, specified type NEC), **M17.11** (Osteoarthritis, knee)

Case 37
Facility: 29877-LT (Arthroscopy, Surgical, Knee), **29874-LT** (Arthroscopy, Surgical, Knee); **996.59** (Complication, mechanical, nonabsorbable surgical material), **716.86** (Arthropathy, specified NEC)

ICD-10-CM: T85.662S (Complication, suture, permanent [wire] NEC, mechanical, displacement), **M12.862** (Arthropathy, specified form NEC, knee)

Case 38
Facility: 25606-LT (Fracture, Radius, Percutaneous Fixation); **813.42** (Fracture, radius, lower end or extremity)

ICD-10-CM: S52.572A (Fracture, traumatic, radius, lower end, intraarticular NEC)

Case 39
Facility: 28124-T9 (Phalanx, Toe, Excision); **733.82** (Nonunion, fracture), **755.66** (Anomaly, toe)

ICD-10-CM: S92.534K (Fracture, traumatic, toe, lesser, distal phalanx, nondisplaced), **Q74.2** (Anomaly, toe)

Case 40
Facility: 29866-RT (Arthroscopy, Surgical, Knee, Osteochondral Autograft); **716.96** (Osteoarthritis)

ICD-10-CM: M17.11 (Osteoarthritis, primary, knee)

Case 41

Facility: 29805-RT (Arthroscopy, Diagnostic, Shoulder), **23430-RT** (Tenodesis, Biceps Tendon, Shoulder); **840.8** (Sprain, shoulder, and arm, upper), **E928.9** (Injury, injured [accidental(ly)] NEC)

ICD-10-CM: S46.111A (Injury, muscle, biceps, long head, strain), **X58.xxxA** (Injury [accidental] NOS)

CHAPTER 7: OTORHINOLARYNGOLOGY

Case 42

Facility: 69436-50 (Tympanostomy); **381.3** (Otitis, media, exudative, chronic)

ICD-10-CM: H65.493 (Otitis, media, nonsuppurative, chronic)

Case 43

Facility: 42145 (Uvula, Excision), **42826** (Tonsillectomy); **327.23** (Apnea, sleep, obstructive), **474.00** (Tonsillitis, chronic), **528.9** (Hypertrophy, uvula)

ICD-10-CM: G47.33 (Apnea, sleep, obstructive), **J35.01** (Tonsillitis, chronic), **K13.79** (Hypertrophy, uvula)

Case 44

Facility: 42145 (Uvula, Excision); **327.23** (Apnea, sleep, obstructive)

ICD-10-CM: G47.33 (Apnea, sleep, obstructive)

Case 45

Facility: 69436-50 (Tympanostomy); **381.3** (Otitis, media, chronic, with effusion), **381.81** (Dysfunction, Eustachian tube), **389.06** (Loss, hearing, conductive [air], bilateral)

ICD-10-CM: H65.493 (Otitis, media, nonsuppurative, chronic), **H69.93** (Disorder, eustachian tube), **H90.0** (Deafness, conductive, bilateral)

Case 46

Facility: 30520 (Septoplasty); **470** (Deviation, septum [acquired] [nasal])

ICD-10-CM: J34.2 (Deviation, septum [nasal] [acquired])

Case 47

Facility: 42821 (Tonsillectomy); **474.02** (Adenoiditis, chronic, with chronic tonsillitis)

ICD-10-CM: J35.03 (Adenoiditis [chronic], with tonsillitis)

Case 48

Facility: 42820 (Tonsillectomy); **474.02** (Adenoiditis, chronic, with chronic tonsillitis)

ICD-10-CM: J35.03 (Adenoiditis [chronic], with tonsillitis)

Case 49

Facility: 69436-50 (Tympanostomy); **381.01** (Otitis, media, acute, serous), **381.10** (Otitis, media, chronic, serous)

ICD-10-CM: H65.03 (Otitis, media, nonsuppurative, acute or subacute, serous), **H65.23** (Otitis, media, nonsuppurative, chronic, serous)

Case 50

Facility: 30520 (Septoplasty), **30140-50** (Turbinate, Excision); **470** (Deformity, nose, septum), **478.0** (Hypertrophy, nasal, turbinate)

ICD-10-CM: J34.2 (Deformity, nose, septum [acquired]), **J34.3** (Hypertrophy, nasal, turbinate)

Case 51

Facility: 31628-RT (Bronchoscopy, Biopsy), **31632-RT** (Bronchoscopy, Biopsy), **31623-RT** (Bronchoscopy, Brushing, Protected Brushing), **31624-RT** (Bronchoscopy, Alveolar Lavage); **518.3** (Infiltrate, pulmonary)

ICD-10-CM: J82 (Infiltrate, pulmonary)

Case 52

Facility: 95807 (Sleep study); **799.02** (Hypoxia), **447.6** (Angiitis), **780.79** (Fatigue)

ICD-10-CM: R09.01 (Hypoxia), **I77.6** (Angiitis), **R53.83** (Fatigue)

Case 53

Facility: 94620 (Pulmonology, Diagnostic, Stress Test, Pulmonary); **786.09** (Dyspnea)

ICD-10-CM: R06.00 (Dyspnea)

Case 54

Facility: 94060 (Pulmonology, Diagnostic, Spirometry), **94375** (Pulmonology, Diagnostic, Flow-Volume Loop), **94720** (Pulmonology, Diagnostic, Carbon Monoxide Diffusion Capacity), **94260** (Pulmonology, Diagnostic, Thoracic Gas Volume); **786.05** (Shortness, breath), **786.07** (Wheezing), **799.02** (Hypoxia)

ICD-10-CM: R06.02 (Shortness, breath), **R06.2** (Wheezing), **R09.01** (Hypoxia)

Case 55

Facility: 32551 (Thoracostomy, Tube), **75989** (Ultrasound, Drainage, Abscess); **511.9** (Effusion, pleura)

ICD-10-CM: J90 (Effusion, pleura)

Case 56

Facility: 31622-RT (Bronchoscopy, Exploration); **518.0** (Collapse, lung)

ICD-10-CM: J98.19 (Collapse, lung [massive])

Case 57
Facility: 93503 (Insertion, Catheter, Cardiac, Flow Directed); **458.9** (Hypotension)

ICD-10-CM: I95.9 (Hypotension)

CHAPTER 8: GENERAL SURGERY

Case 58
Facility: 54150 (Circumcision, Surgical Excision, Newborn); **605** (Phimosis)

ICD-10-CM: N47.1 (Phimosis)

Case 59
Facility: 52000 (Cystoscopy); **625.6** (Incontinence, urine, stress [female])

ICD-10-CM: N39.3 (Incontinence, urine, stress [female])

Case 60
Facility: 49505-LT (Repair, Hernia, Reducible, Inguinal); **550.90** (Hernia, inguinal [indirect])

ICD-10-CM: K40.90 (Hernia, inguinal [indirect])

Case 61
Facility: 49422 (Removal, Catheter, Peritoneum); **996.68** (Complication, dialysis, catheter, infection or inflammation, peritoneal)

ICD-10-CM: T85.71xA (Complication, catheter, intraperitoneal dialysis, infection and inflammation)

Case 62
Facility: 49422 (Removal, Catheter, Peritoneum), **49421** (Insertion, Catheter, Abdomen); **996.56** (Complication, mechanical, catheter, dialysis, peritoneal), **585.6** (Disease, renal, end-stage), **V45.11** (Status, dialysis [peritoneal])

ICD-10-CM: T85.611A (Complication, catheter, intraperitoneal dialysis, mechanical breakdown, initial encounter), **N18.6** (Failure, renal, end stage [chronic]), **Z99.2** (Status, dialysis [peritoneal])

Case 63
Facility: 43262 (Cholangiopancreatography, with Surgery); **789.00** (Pain, abdominal, unspecified), **790.5** (Findings, abnormal, without diagnosis, enzymes, serum)

ICD-10-CM: R10.9 (Pain, abdominal, unspecified), **R74.8** (Abnormal, serum level [of], enzymes, specified NEC)

Case 64
Facility: 47562 (Laparoscopy, Cholecystectomy); **574.30** (Choledocholithiasis, with, cholecystitis, acute)

ICD-10-CM: K80.42 (Calculus, bile duct, with cholecystis [with cholangitis], acute)

Case 65
Facility: 38542-RT (Lymph Nodes, Dissection); **785.6** (Lymphadenopathy [general])

ICD-10-CM: R59.0 (Lymphadenopathy, localized)

Case 66
Facility: 38221 (Bone Marrow, Needle Biopsy); **284.9** (Anemia, aplastic), **202.80** (Lymphoma, unspecified site)

ICD-10-CM: D61.9 (Anemia, aplastic), **C85.90** (Lymphoma [malignant])

CHAPTER 9: EMERGENCY DEPARTMENT

Case 67
Professional Services: 99282 (Evaluation and Management, Emergency Department); **847.0** (Sprain, neck), **E819.1** (Accident, motor vehicle, Passenger in motor vehicle)

Facility Services: 99282 (Level 2, Point 6); **847.0** (Sprain, neck), **E819.1** (Accident, motor vehicle, Passenger in motor vehicle)

ICD-10-CM: S13.4xxA (Sprain, neck, cervical spine), **V49.9xxA** (Accident, transport, car occupant)

Case 68
Professional Services: 99283 (Evaluation and Management, Emergency Department); **724.2** (Pain, low back), **564.00** (Constipation)

Facility Services: 99283 (Level 3, Point 3); **724.2** (Pain, low back), **564.00** (Constipation, unspecified)

ICD-10-CM: M54.5 (Pain, low back), **K59.00** (Constipation, unspecified)

Case 69
Professional Services: 99285 (Evaluation and Management, Emergency Department); **786.50** (Pain, chest [central], unspecified), **285.9** (Anemia, unspecified)

Facility Services: This is an inpatient stay. The entire record would need to be reviewed before coding. We will not be assigning codes on inpatients. The facility charges for the emergency department visit would be included on the inpatient billing.

ICD-10-CM: R07.9 (Pain, chest (central), unspecified), **D64.9** (Anemia, unspecified)

Case 70
Professional Services: 99283 (Evaluation and Management, Emergency Department); **893.0** (Wound, open, toe[s] [nail]), **924.3** (Contusion, toe[s] [nail] [subungual]), **E916** (Hit by, object, falling)

Facility Services: 99283 (Level 3, Point 3); **893.0** (Wound, open, toe(s), [nail]), **924.3** (Contusion, toe[s] [nail] [subungual]), **E916** (Hit [accidental] by, object, falling)

ICD-10-CM: S91.205A (Wound, open, toe[s], lesser, left, with damage to the nail), **S90.122A** (Contusion, toe[s] [lesser]), **S90.222A** (Contusion, toe[s] [lesser], with damage to nail), **W20.8xxA** (Struck by, object, falling)

Case 71
Facility Services: 12032 (Repair, Skin, Wound, Intermediate); **891.0** (Wound, open, leg, lower), **E916** (Hit, hitting by, object, falling)

ICD-10-CM: S81.811A (Laceration, leg [lower]), **W20.8xxA** (Hit, hitting by, object, falling, initial encounter)

Case 72
Professional Services: 99283 (Evaluation and Management, Emergency Department); **789.04** (Pain, abdominal, left lower quadrant), **787.91** (Diarrhea)

Facility Services: 99383 (Level 3, Points 3 and 10); **789.04** (Pain, abdomen, left lower quadrant), **787.91** (Diarrhea)

ICD-10-CM: R10.32 (Pain, abdomen, lower, left quadrant), **R19.7** (Diarrhea)

Case 73
Professional Services: 99283 (Evaluation and Management, Emergency Department); **784.0** (Headache), **780.60** (Fever, with chills)

Facility Services: 99283 (Level 3, Point 4); **784.0** (Headache), **780.60** (Fever, with chills)

ICD-10-CM: R51 (Headache), **R50.9** (Fever [with chills])

Case 74
Professional Services: 99285 (Evaluation and Management, Emergency Department); **486** (Pneumonia), **799.02** (Hypoxia)

Facility Services: This is an inpatient stay. The entire record would need to be reviewed before coding. We will not be assigning codes on inpatients. The facility charges for the emergency department visit would be included on the inpatient billing.

ICD-10-CM: J18.9 (Pneumonia), **R09.01** (Hypoxia)

Case 75
Professional Services: 99282 (Evaluation and Management, Emergency Department), **599.71** (Hematuria, gross)

Facility Services: 99282 (Level 2, Point 3), **599.71** (Hematuria, gross)

ICD-10-CM: R31.0 (Hematuria, gross)

Case 76
Professional Services: 99285 (Evaluation and Management, Emergency Department); **805.2** (Fracture, vertebra, thoracic [closed]), **V15.51** (History [personal], fracture, healed, traumatic), **E888.9** (Fall, falling, same level NEC), **E849.0** (Accident, occurring [in], residence, home [private]), **E001.0** (Activity [involving], walking [on level or elevated terrain])

Facility Services: This is an inpatient stay. The entire record would need to be reviewed before coding. We will not be assigning codes on inpatients. The facility charges for the emergency department visit would be included on the inpatient billing.

ICD-10-CM: S22.030A (Fracture, traumatic, thorax, vertebra, third, wedge compression), **S22.060A** (Fracture, traumatic, thorax, vertebra, eighth, wedge compression), **Z87.81** (History, personal [of], fracture [healed], traumatic), **W18.30xA** (Fall, falling, same level), **Y92.00** (Place of occurrence, residence), **Y93.01** (Activity, walking [on level or elevated terrain])

CHAPTER 10: DIAGNOSTIC RADIOLOGY

Case 77
Facility: 93880 (Duplex Scan, Arterial Studies, Extracranial); **433.10** (Narrowing, artery, carotid, without mention of cerebral infarction)

ICD-10-CM: I65.21 (Occlusion, artery, carotid)

Case 78
Facility: 76830 (Echography, Transvaginal), **76856** (Echography, Pelvis); **625.8** (Cramp[s], uterus)

ICD-10-CM: N94.89 (Cramp[s], uterus)

Case 79
Facility: 76770 (Echography, Retroperitoneal); **585.9** (Disease, kidney, chronic, unspecified stage)

ICD-10-CM: N18.9 (Disease, kidney, chronic)

Case 80
Facility: 76816 (Ultrasound, Pregnant Uterus); **644.03** (Labor, premature, threatened)

ICD-10-CM: O60.03 (Pregnancy, complicated by, preterm labor, third trimester, without delivery)

Case 81
Facility: 76820 (Ultrasound, Umbilical Artery); **642.93** (Hypertension, complicating pregnancy, childbirth, or the puerperium, unspecified)

ICD-10-CM: O10.913 (Hypertension, complicating pregnancy, pre-existing)

Case 82
Facility: 76818 (Ultrasound, Fetus); **655.73** (Decrease, fetal movements, antepartum)

ICD-10-CM: O36.8190 (Pregnancy, complicated by, decreased fetal movements)

Case 83
Facility: 76705 (Echography, Abdomen); **575.8** (Distension, distention, gallbladder)

ICD-10-CM: K82.8 (Distention, gallbladder)

Case 84
Facility: 73700-RT (CT Scan, without Contrast, Leg); **996.62** (Complications, infection and inflammation, due to any device, implant, or graft, catheter, vascular)

ICD-10-CM: T82.7xxA (Complications, extremity artery [bypass] graft, infection and inflammation)

Case 85
Facility: 71260 (CT Scan, with Contrast, Thorax); **511.9** (Effusion, pleura), **492.0** (Emphysema, bullous), **V45.81** (Status [post], aortocoronary bypass)

ICD-10-CM: J90 (Effusion, pleura), **J43.9** (Emphysema [bullous]), **Z95.1** (Status [post], aortocoronary bypass or shunt)

Case 86
Facility: 70450 (CT Scan, without Contrast, Brain); **784.0** (Headache)

ICD-10-CM: R51 (Headache)

Case 87
Facility: 70491 (CT Scan, with Contrast, Neck); **785.6** (Hypertrophy, lymph gland)

ICD-10-CM: R59.0 (Hypertrophy, lymph, lymphatic gland, localized)

Case 88
Facility: 70491 (CT Scan, with Contrast, Neck); **787.20** (Dysphagia), **784.2** (Swelling, neck)

ICD-10-CM: R13.10 (Dysphagia), **R22.1** (Swelling, localized [skin], neck)

Case 89
Facility: 70486 (CT Scan, without Contrast, Face); **473.9** (Sinusitis, chronic)

ICD-10-CM: J32.9 (Sinusitis, chronic)

Case 90
Facility: 73718-LT (Magnetic Resonance Imaging, (MRI), Foot); **682.7** (Cellulitis, foot [except toes])

ICD-10-CM: L03.116 (Cellulitis, lower limb)

Case 91
Facility: 74185 (Magnetic Resonance Angiography, Abdomen); **403.90** (Hypertension, with, chronic kidney disease, stage 1 through stage IV, or unspecified), **585.9** (Disease, kidney, chronic), **710.0** (Lupus)

ICD-10-CM: I12.9 (Hypertension, with, kidney disease, stage I through stage IV, chronic kidney disease), **N18.9** (Disease, kidney, chronic), **M32.9** (Lupus, systemic)

Case 92
Facility: 73218-F3 (Magnetic Resonance Imaging, (MRI), Hand), **681.00** (Cellulitis, finger)

ICD-10-CM: L03.012 (Cellulitis, finger, left)

Case 93
Facility: 70553 (Magnetic Resonance Imaging, (MRI), Brain); **784.59** (Slurred, slurring, speech), **728.87** (Weak, muscle, generalized)

ICD-10-CM: R47.81 (Slurred, slurring, speech), **M62.81** (Weak, muscle)

Case 94
Facility: 93922 (Doppler Scan, Arterial Studies, Extremities); **443.9** (Insufficiency, arterial, peripheral)

ICD-10-CM: I73.9 (Insufficiency, arterial, peripheral)

Case 95
Facility: 71010 (X-ray, Chest); **441.9** (Aneurysm, aortic)

ICD-10-CM: I71.9 (Aneurysm, aortic)

Case 96
Facility: 74230 (Pharynx, Video Study); **787.20** (Dysphagia)

ICD-10-CM: R13.10 (Dysphagia)

Case 97
Facility: 74020 (X-Ray, Abdomen); **789.00** (Pain, abdominal)

ICD-10-CM: R10.9 (Pain, abdominal)

CHAPTER 11: INTERVENTIONAL RADIOLOGY, RADIATION ONCOLOGY, AND NUCLEAR MEDICINE

Case 98
Facility: 20206-RT (Biopsy, Muscle), **77012** (CT Scan, Guidance, Needle Placement); **686.9** (Inflammation, subcutaneous tissue), **718.35** (Dislocation, hip, recurrent)

ICD-10-CM: L08.9 (Inflammation, subcutaneous tissue), **M24.451** (Dislocation, recurrent, hip, right)

Case 99
Facility: 36569 (Catheterization, Peripheral); **709.8** (Necrosis, skin or subcutaneous tissue)

ICD-10-CM: I96 (Necrosis, skin or subcutaneous tissue NEC)

Case 100
Facility: 36558 (Catheterization, Central), **77001** (Venous Access Device, Fluoroscopic Guidance); **585.9** (Disease, kidney, chronic)

ICD-10-CM: N18.9 (Disease, kidney, chronic)

Case 101
Facility: 174.2 (Neoplasm, breast, upper-inner quadrant, Malignant, Primary), **196.3** (Neoplasm, lymph, gland, axillary, Malignant, Secondary). The facility would not bill for treatment planning (77263) as that is only a professional service.

ICD-10-CM: C50.212 (Neoplasm, breast, female, upper-inner quadrant, left, Malignant Primary), **C77.3** (Neoplasm, lymph, gland, axilla, axillary, Malignant Secondary)

Case 102
Facility: 77295 (Radiation Therapy, Field Set-Up); **174.2** (Neoplasm, breast, upper-inner quadrant, Malignant, Primary), **196.3** (Neoplasm, lymph, gland, axillary, Malignant, Secondary)

ICD-10-CM: C50.212 (Neoplasm, breast, female, upper-inner quadrant, Malignant Primary), **C77.3** (Neoplasm, lymph, gland, axillary, Malignant Secondary)

Case 103
Facility: 77785 (Brachytherapy, Remote Afterloading, 1 Channel); **414.02** (Arteriosclerosis, bypass graft, coronary artery, autologous vein), **V45.81** (Status, coronary artery bypass or shunt)

ICD-10-CM: I25.810 (Arteriosclerosis, coronary artery, bypass graft, autologous vein), **Z95.1** (Status, aortocoronary bypass)

Case 104
Facility: 78452 (Nuclear Medicine, Heart, Myocardial Perfusion); **786.05** (Shortness, breath), **V45.01** (Status [post], pacemaker, cardiac)

ICD-10-CM: R06.02 (Shortness, breath), **Z95.0** (Status [post], pacemaker, cardiac)

Case 105
Facility: 78452 (Nuclear Medicine, Heart, Myocardial Perfusion); **786.50** (Pain, chest)

ICD-10-CM: R07.9 (Pain, chest [central])

CHAPTER 12: CARDIOLOGY

Case 106
Facility: 92960 (Cardioversion); **427.31** (Fibrillation, atrial)

ICD-10-CM: I48.0 (Fibrillation, atrial or auricular NEC)

Case 107
Facility: 93017 (Exercise Stress Test, Tracing); **412** (History, personal [of], myocardial infarction), **V45.82** (Status [post], angioplasty, percutaneous transluminal, coronary)

ICD-10-CM: I25.2 (History, personal [of], myocardial infarction [old]), **Z95.5** (Status [post], angioplasty, coronary artery, with implant)

Case 108
Facility: 93308 (Echocardiography, Cardiac, Transthoracic), **93321** (Echocardiography, Cardiac, Doppler), **93325** (Echocardiography, Cardiac); **428.0** (Failure, heart, congestive)

ICD-10-CM: I50.9 (Failure, heart, congestive)

Case 109
Facility: 93017 (Exercise Stress Test, tracing); **414.01** (Arteriosclerosis, coronary [artery], native artery), **V45.01** (Status [post], pacemaker, cardiac)

ICD-10-CM: I25.10 (Arteriosclerosis, coronary [artery]), **Z95.0** (Status [post], pacemaker, cardiac)

Case 110
Facility: 93017 (Exercise Stress Test, tracing); **412** (Infarction, myocardium, healed or old, currently presenting no symptoms), **V45.81** (Status [post], coronary artery bypass or shunt), **V45.01** (Status [post], pacemaker, cardiac)

ICD-10-CM: I25.2 (History, personal [of], myocardial infarction [old]), **Z95.1** (Status [post], aortocoronary bypass), **Z95.0** (Status [post], pacemaker, cardiac)

Case 111
Facility: 93460 (Cardiac, Catheterization, Combined Left and Right); **425.4** (Cardiomyopathy), **414.01** (Arteriosclerosis, coronary [artery], native artery), **416.8** (Hypertension, pulmonary, Unspecified), **794.39** (Findings, abnormal, without diagnosis, stress test)

ICD-10-CM: I42.9 (Cardiomyopathy), **I25.10** (Arteriosclerosis, coronary [artery], native artery), **I27.2** (Hypertension, pulmonary [artery] [secondary] NEC), **R94.39** (Findings, abnormal, inconclusive, without diagnosis, stress test)

Case 112
Facility: 93458 (Cardiac Catheterization, Left Heart); **794.39** (Findings, abnormal, stress test), **784.92** (Pain[s], jaw), **401.9** (Hypertension)

ICD-10-CM: R94.39 (Findings, abnormal, inconclusive, without diagnosis, stress test), **M27.8** (Pain, jaw), **I10** (Hypertension)

CHAPTER 13: INPATIENT CASES

Case 113
Facility: 821.23 (Fracture, femur, femoral, supracondylar), **285.9** (Anemia), **496** (Disease, pulmonary, obstructive diffuse [chronic]), **V58.65** (Long-term [current], drug use, steroids), **V46.2** (Dependence [on], supplemental oxygen), **E888.9** (Fall, falling, same level NEC), **E849.0** (Accident, occurring [at], home); **79.35** (Reduction, fracture, femur, open, with internal fixation), **99.04** (Transfusion, packed cells)

ICD-10-CM: S72.452A (Fracture, traumatic, femur, lower end, supracondylar [displaced]), **D64.9** (Anemia), **J44.9** (Disease, pulmonary, chronic, obstructive), **Z79.52** (Long, term [current], drug therapy, steroids, systemic), **Z99.81** (Dependence on, oxygen [long-term] [supplemental]), **W18.30xA** (Fall, same level NEC), **Y92.00** (Place of occurrence, residence [private])

Case 114
Facility: 820.21 (Fracture, femur, femoral, neck, intertrochanteric), **780.39** (Seizure), **250.41** (Diabetes, with, nephropathy), **583.81** (Nephropathy, diabetic), **585.6** (Disease, renal, end-stage), **403.91** (Hypertension, with, stage V or end stage renal disease), **250.61** (Diabetes, with, gastroparesis), **536.3** (Gastroparesis), **205.00** (Leukemia, myelogenous, acute, without mention of having achieved remission), **V42.0** (Status [post], transplant, kidney), **V58.65** (Long-term [current] drug use, insulin), **V45.11** (Dependence, on, renal dialysis machine), **E885.9** (Fall, falling, same level from slipping, stumbling, tripping), **E849.0** (Accident, occurring [at], home); **81.52** (Arthroplasty, hip, femoral head, with prosthetic implant), **39.95** (Dialysis, hemodiafiltration, hemofiltration [extracorporeal])

ICD-10-CM: S72.142A (Fracture, traumatic, femur, trochanteric, intertrochanteric [displaced]), **R56.9** (Seizure), **E10.21** (Diabetes, type I, with nephropathy), **N18.6** (Disease, renal, end-stage), **I12.0** (Hypertension, with, kidney, with, stage V chronic kidney disease [CKD] or end stage renal disease [ESRD]), **E10.43** (Diabetes, diabetic, type 1, with, gastroparesis), **C92.00** (Leukemia, myelogenous), **Z94.0** (Transplant, kidney), **Z79.4** (Long, term [current] drug therapy, insulin), **Z99.2** (Dependence, on, renal dialysis [hemodialysis]), **W01.0xxA** (Fall, falling, same level, from, slipping, stumbling, tripping), **Y92.00** (Place of occurrence, residence [private])

Case 115
Facility: 584.9 (Failure, renal, acute), **593.3** (Stricture/Stenosis, ureter), **275.41** (Hypocalcemia), **275.2** (Hypomagnesemia), **275.3** (Hypophosphatemia), **276.2** (Acidosis), **591** (Hydronephrosis), **174.9** (Neoplasm, breast, Malignant, Primary), **198.5** (Neoplasm, spine, Malignant, Secondary), **198.89** (Neoplasm, abdominal cavity, Malignant, Secondary), **285.29** (Anemia, in, chronic illness NEC), **263.9** (Malnutrition), **298.9** (Confusion, confused), **785.6** (Lymphadenopathy), **338.4** (Pain, chronic, syndrome); **57.32** (Cystoscopy, transurethral), **59.8** (Insertion, ureteral stent)

ICD-10-CM: N17.9 (Failure, renal, acute), **N13.1** (Stricture, ureter, with, hydronephrosis), **E83.51** (Hypocalcemia), **E83.42** (Hypomagnesemia), **E83.39** (Hypophosphatemia), **E87.2** (Acidosis), **C50.912** (Neoplasm, breast, female, unspecified site, left side, Malignant Primary), **C79.51** (Neoplasm, spine, Malignant Secondary), **C79.89** (Neoplasm, abdominal cavity, Malignant Secondary), **D63.8** (Anemia, due to, chronic disease classified elsewhere), **E46** (Malnutrition), **F44.89** (State [of] confusional), **R59.0** (Lymphadenopathy, localized), **R52** (Pain, chronic)

Case 116
Facility: 733.19 (Fracture, pathologic, specified site), **585.6** (Disease, renal, end-stage), **250.01** (Diabetes, type I), **276.1** (Hyponatremia), **276.8** (Hypokalemia), **288.60** (Leukocytosis), **443.9** (Disease, vascular, peripheral), **V58.61** (Long-term drug use, anticoagulants), **787.01** (Nausea, with vomiting), **V58.67** (Long-term [current], drug, insulin); **54.98** (Dialysis, peritoneal), **88.26** (Radiography, pelvis [skeletal]), **92.18** (Scan, scanning, radioisotope, total bone)

ICD-10-CM: M84.454A (Fracture, pathologic, pelvis), **N18.6** (Disease, renal, end-stage [failure]), **E10.9** (Diabetes, type I), **E87.1** (Hyponatremia), **E87.6** (Hypokalemia), **D72.829** (Leukocytosis), **I73.9** (Disease, vascular, peripheral [occlusive]), **Z79.01** (Long, term [current] drug therapy, anticoagulants), **R11.2** (Nausea, with vomiting), **Z79.4** (Long-term [current] drug therapy, insulin)

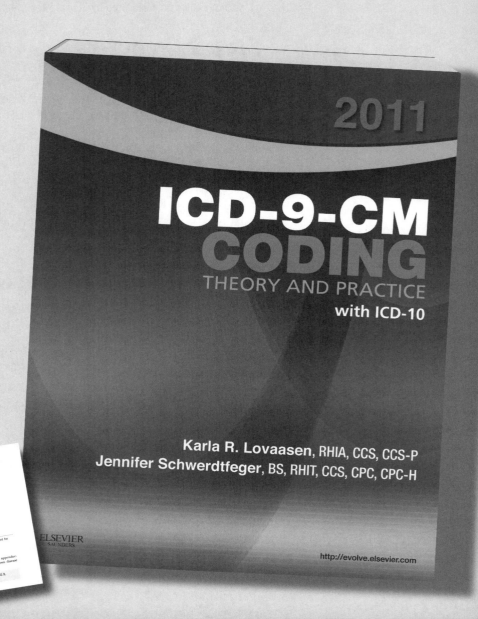

Trust Carol J. Buck and Elsevier for the

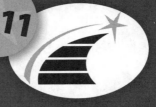

resources you need at *each step* of your coding career!

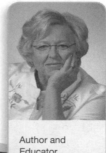